Digital Minimalism

How to Overcome Technology Addiction.

A 10 Steps Program to Declutter Your Digital Life, Live with Less Distraction, Stay Focused, and Regain Your Freedom

Mark Ernest Johnson

Introduction   **5**

Chapter 1: The Social Networks Era: How They Impact Our Life   **8**

Health   10

Emotional   10

Communication   11

Tech-Savvy Parents   12

Why Our Screens Make Us Less Happy   15

Getting Notification Constantly Kills Your Productivity 18

Easier to Change Your Bad Habits Than Quitting Cold Turkey   19

Chapter 2: How We Became Digital Zombies   **22**

Rethinking Your Relationship With Your Phone   27

FOMO and Phubbing   30

Learning to Control Your Addiction   34

Chapter 3: How Your Brain Is Getting Hacked: The Evil Side of Social Networks   **38**

Your Cell Phone Is a Slot Machine   41

Likes Are The New Nicotine   53

Social Networks Manipulate Your Brain   58

It's All Engineered   69

Chapter 4: How They Manipulate Your Brain: The Vegas Effect and Desire for Social Approval   **78**

Vegas Effect and Intermittent Reinforcement Schedules80

Our Need for Approval   89

Chapter 5: Impact of Social Networks in Our Democracies   **98**

Cambridge Analytica   98

Russia's Cyberwarfare   104

Russia's Interference With the 2016 US Elections   110

Russian's Interference With the US 2018 Elections   113

Russia's Interference With the 2016 Brexit Referendum114

Russian's Intelligence Agencies Send Misinformation About COVID-19   117

Coronavirus False Information and Ways Scientists Can Fight It   125

Chapter 6: Digital Minimalism and Digital Detox   **133**

10-Steps to a Digital Detox   134

Quitting Social Media   149

Digital Declutter   156

Practices   159

Social Media Contradiction   166

Reclaiming Conversations   167

Reclaim Your Leisure Time   169

Tech Could Protect Us   171

Conclusion   **173**

Introduction

First off, I would like to thank you for choosing this book, and I hope that it is able to guide you through the world of digital minimalism to help make your life healthier.

The purpose of this book is to help you realize the dangers of excessive social media use. Social networks are not as innocent as they seem, and they definitely have grown way beyond what they were created for. They have developed a psychological hold on us that nobody realized would happen. Now, some people realize that this hold has developed, and they are using it to take advantage of us.

This has caused a brand new addiction. Social networks create the same response in our brain as alcohol, drugs, and nicotine does, and that's why you feel that need, that itch, to check your notifications. Every time your phone goes off, you jump with anticipation for what it says. This is not healthy and can have serious negative consequences on your health.

That's what leads us to our first chapter, where we will look at the impact social networks have on our lives. Social media, as we know it, has only been around for just about two decades, but it has created deep roots in our psyche, and it is crucial to understand how this affects us.

Then we will move into discussing the addiction we have developed for our smartphones. We have all been turned into digital zombies, so much so that we often neglect human connection in order to get our next like. We'll look at the importance of rethinking the relationship we have with our phones and how we can deal with FOMO.

Next is probably the most important thing that we need to talk about. It is a fact that social media has become the nicotine. We have little control over social media, and this did not happen by accident. All of the ads and shiny things in and on social media have been placed there to grab our attention and pull us in.

To expand on that addiction, we will go over how exactly social media manipulates the brain by looking at the Vegas effect and the need for approval. These are all the psychological effects that people who run social media use to their advantage.

After that, we will take a look at how social media is affecting our government and democracy. We are all very aware of the Russian Cyberwarfare problem that happened during the last election. Then there is also the issue of fake news that continues to grow. That means not only does social media affects our minds, but it allows people to outright lie, but convince others that it is the truth.

Lastly, we will wrap things up by talking about digital minimalism and how to go through a digital detox. The only way to stop the damage from social media is to stop using it for a little while. You don't have to give it up altogether, but it does not hurt to take a step away and get rid of the addiction. After that, you will need to pay attention to your social media use, and any digital use, to make sure that you don't fall into its trap again.

Before we begin, I would like to ask that if you find any part of this book helpful, in any way, please leave a review. Let's begin.

Chapter 1: The Social Networks Era: How They Impact Our Life

Parents today have the impression that computers are our future, and everybody, even young children, need to be computer savvy as soon as they can be. If you follow this theory, failing to expose our children to technology will keep them from being able to function in the world.

BUT, getting addicted to every present tiny screen could be the real handicap. Not exposing our children to technology may be more of an advantage in today's completely connected world.

Social media has been having a huge impact on our lives. Even though having some exposure to social media could be positive, it has shown to have a negative effect on things like our stress levels and moods. You can be addicted to social media, too. Since we have access to it all day long on our phones, it is easy to get into a bad habit of checking it almost constantly. We check it while listening to a professor while eating, or even when we go to bed. Here are some areas where being addicted to social media can have negative impacts.

Health

Since you can become addicted to social media, it can affect our sleep. Using any kind of electronic devices such as video games or cell phones right before you go to bed can cause various sleep problems. This could then lead to other problems like falling asleep in class, while driving, or not being able to focus because they are too tired.

Emotional

Several studies have shown that using social media can cause have a negative impact on mental health, bad moods, and stress. Most people wake up each morning and immediately reach for their phones to check their Twitter, Snapchat, Instagram, or Facebook. With platforms such as Instagram, users feel like they are obligated to edit a post so that it fits into the "attractiveness" terms. Users might start comparing themselves to other users and think: "Am I pretty enough?" "Am I good enough?"

Communication

Before texting was invented, when you wanted to get in touch with someone, you had to call them. Even though electronic messaging does make communications more accessible and faster, there could be negative impacts of it, too. It is tricky to figure out someone's tone when they are using social media or texting.

Social media can be compelling. It helps people all over the world to connect, and it inspires people to reach social change. We have to also realize all the negative impacts that it can have on our lives. We don't need social media in our waking lives. You have to realize that you need to work on your relationship in real-time and not just through a screen.

Tech-Savvy Parents

These views aren't ones of parents who are being overprotective or parents who aren't familiar with the technology. The biggest promoters of computer gadgets have been known to discourage the products that they make. The best example is the co-founder of Apple, Steve Jobs. He claimed that he didn't allow his children to have iPads, iPhones, or iPods, and he also limited how long they were allowed to use technology when home.

In 2010 when iPads exploded onto the markets, Jobs' daughters Eve and Erin were not a part of this market. Jobs, along with his wife Laurene Powell, regulated how much their daughters were exposed to this new product.

What did the girls do rather than surf the web or texting? Well, they did all the things that normal children are supposed to do. The family ate dinner together each night. They talked about history, books, and other things that had nothing to do with technology. Devices like iPhones, iPads, or other

13

technology were never allowed to be at their table. Their children didn't seem to be bothered by this.

Jobs thought that by limiting their computer use would help them have a love for creativity. He didn't want them wasting their time on useless programs and games. This was completely opposite of his job to fill the world with gadgets that changed how people would communicate, entertain themselves, and listen to music. The things he marketed toward others, he didn't want for his children.

Steve Jobs wasn't alone in his thinking. There is a large number of tech executives that limit how much exposure their children had to all the technology they were producing, designing, and marketing. These parents said the attraction of the new technology was overwhelming and children's addiction to these factored into their decisions.

An example of this trend can be found at an elementary school in Silicon Valley. Many executives and engineers from tech companies such as Yahoo, Hewlett-Packard, Google, eBay, and Apple enroll their children in a

Waldorf school located in Los Altos, California. Electronic devices aren't allowed, and neither is watching television. They state that these radical measures are needed to make sure children develop all of their talents without distractions.

These so-called radical measures aren't all that radical. Parents don't have to send their children to private schools that are expensive to give their children the same advantages as the Waldorf School.

All any parent needs to do is to allow their children to be a child. Children need to be allowed to grow up as a child with all the spontaneity, creativity, and interaction that will always be a part of a healthy childhood. They need to be allowed to play games, eat as a family, and solve their problems together.

The true radicals are the parents who let their children be tethered to their devices and never learning how to be part of the real world. If you have any doubts about this, just keep reading.

Why Our Screens Make Us Less Happy

You are probably reading this book from a device. And you have likely picked it up more times today than you even realize. Everybody shared on social media; we check our notifications. So, what is wrong with being connected in life?

The biggest problem with being constantly linked to technology is that we can become addicted to it. You might say that we think of them as irresistible.

Even though tablets, smartphones, and other devices have made our lives a lot more convenient, they have come at a cost. This price is we are missing opportunities to experience and connect with life on the deepest levels possible.

You might be thinking that you don't have a problem, but most of us will check our phones a lot more than we realize. If you don't think there is any harm in all of this, keep reading to find out why you are wrong.

Here are three huge lessons about smartphone addiction that you probably didn't know:

Smartphone Addiction and Drug Addiction are Very Similar

When I mention the word addiction, you probably think of alcohol or drug addiction. Scientists are finding that certain activities that we do often can affect our brains the same way severe addictions can.

In every case, our bodies release dopamine. This will signal intense pleasures in our brains. The bigger problem is the enjoyment that we get from these actions decrease every time we do it.

If you are trying to achieve that high from scrolling through social media, you are just looking for more and more pleasure. The dopamine that gets released gets smaller the more you scroll through your feed. This, in turn, creates a habit or an addiction.

17

Even though you may not see it, all the negative side effects are there. Lack of sleep is the best example I can give you. The light that our phones emit tells our bodies that it is still daytime, and we need to remain awake. If we use them before we go to bed, it programs our minds that our bed is a place where we need to be awake and not sleep.

The good news is that although our addictions to electronic devices are, in fact, similar to drug addiction, these will be easier to break since they aren't as intense.

Getting Notification Constantly Kills Your Productivity

A few seconds ago, while writing this book, I got a notification on my phone from Facebook. Without even thinking about it, I opened it to see if it was something important. Before I realized what was happening, ten minutes had passed. If it wasn't for my computer screen going to sleep, I might not have gotten back to this book at all today.

Research has shown that about 70 percent of all emails get read in just a few seconds. This makes us think that we are very productive, but the truth is that it is the total opposite. Anytime we get a notification, we think we have to stop. It is estimated that it will take us 25 minutes to get back to work.

This means that any employee who checks their email an average of 25 times each day they won't ever get focused entirely on their work. Ues, we feel good when we check our emails quickly because we think we are winning, but it comes at a cost that is a lot higher.

We need to turn off all notifications on your computer, phone, and other devices. Create a specific time where you can check and respond to your emails. When people are forced not to check their email for a period of time will actually experience several benefits. They get out and enjoy nature, the interaction with others, and walk. Research has shown that the more we focus

19

longer means we will be more productive because we aren't checking our emails as often.

Easier to Change Your Bad Habits Than Quitting Cold Turkey

Try to think of a habit that you are trying to quit. Have you tried to stop it more than one time? Many people end up trying to break their bad habits by going cold turkey. Typically, this just leaves us feeling frustrated and starting it all over again. There is a better way to do it.

Rather than attempting to sever all ties with your addiction, try to substitute it for a better habit. There is a thing known as a "habit loop" that can be broken into three parts:

- Your cue

- Your routine

- Your reward

Every one of these will be present anytime you pick up your smartphone. Your cue is picking up your phone. Your routine is opening up an app. Your reward is feeling connected and getting likes. You can change these patterns and get some benefits.

If you have decided you want to have a better relationship with technology, you have to replace your routine in the habit loop. Rather than grabbing your phone, try picking up a book or other things you used to enjoy having in your hands. Do this each day for a week, and you will see that your fitness, mental health, and relationships have improved.

Chapter 2: How We Became Digital Zombies

Every day of our life, technology takes over more and more. Regardless of your economic status, career, ethnicity, gender, or age, you likely have a smartphone. 56% of all Americans own one. Tablets, computers, and phones have transitioned away from being just devices and into being the best friend to many.

There are those people who experience anxiety when they can't find their phones, even if it is only for a few minutes. We all rely on our phones to do so much for us, from saying "I love you" to checking our bank account. We can use our phones to help us with a plethora of tasks, and they fit right in the palm of our hands.

This shouldn't come as a surprise. Just take a look at when and where you use your phone. Are you on it while eating dinner? It's normal to look across the dinner table to see your sibling, parent, or partner checking the texts, updates, tweets, or emails. Even in a dark theater, where phones are supposed to be silences, you can see the glow of the light coming from several seats. Women used to head to the Ladies' Room in pairs, but now they have started to take their phone instead. Men do this, as well.

Our phones have become such a problem that people still think that they can text and drive. Parents use their phones during the children's performances, and not to record them. Then there is the fact that so many people use their phone while having an in-person conversation with somebody. It's rude and disrespectful, but we don't see it that way anymore.

What's worse, Americans have started to bring their phone into bed with them. They are not texting while having sex. There was a survey done, and of those who replied, one in ten admitted to using their phone during sex. When it comes to those aged 18 to 34, that becomes one in five.

That's not the worst fact about cell phone addiction. 50% of people surveyed by Mobile Consumer Habits said that they have texted while driving even though it has been proven that it is six times more dangerous than drunk driving.

Do we really need to post, text, talk, and tweet while we have sex or take a shower? This "I have to have my phone at all times" mindset has become a huge problem. There has even been a name coined for this fear of being without your phone, nomophobia. Nomophobia is characterized by that rush of fear and anxiety when you realize that you aren't connected within your loop of friends and family.

This disconnect can happen in different ways. You can experience when you lose connection, have a dead battery, run out of minutes, forget your phone, or, and this is the worst one, lost your phone. It's probably safe to say that many of you had a lurch in your stomach just by reading those words.

Before you think this is only a US issue, it's not. According to Vesapak, 41% of Britons feel worried, anxious, or out of control when they don't have their tablet o smartphone, and 51% have said that they suffer from "extreme tech anxiety."

We view the phone as an extension of ourselves, so the loss can feel similar to how it feels to lose a best friend. Another interesting thing is that not have a phone connection is social in nature. This means that it isn't important that your boss wants you to be in by 10, but it is vital to know that Katy Perry just had her baby. That makes it a lot less surprising to find out that 75% of people have said that their phones are less than five feet from them at all times.

Pretty much anything in life can be abused, including the phone. As we grow even more tech-savvy and tech-hungry, creating phone-free zones is going to become more common. Think about the fact that smoking use to be allowed and even encouraged on flights. But as smoking gained hostility for its ill-effects on our health, smoke-free zones started to pop up everywhere.

If you still don't believe you could be addicted to your cell phone, here are some symptoms:

1. Anxiety – When you don't have your phone

within arm's length, you start to feel anxious.

2. Constantly checking – You are always checking your phone for new texts, along with the need to respond immediately.

3. False buzz – You feel as if your phone just vibrated, yet when you check the phone, and there is nothing there. This is a real syndrome known as phantom cellphone vibration syndrome.

4. You don't listen – You don't listen to what others are saying, and you couldn't even repeat back what the person in front of you just said. You can't because you have been scrolling through Facebook.

5. Failing – Getting low grades can often be the cause of smartphone   use in class.

6. Turning around – You are on the way to the

store, or somewhere else, and 30 minutes into the trip, you realize you forgot your phone, and you have to turn around to get it.

If continually checking your phone comes as natural as breathing, or you feel restless and anxious when you can't easily reach your phone, you likely have an addiction.

Rethinking Your Relationship With Your Phone

Think about all of the time that you spend on your phone, and what you could be doing if you weren't on your phone. The average person spends three hours and 15 minutes. That's a lot of time that could be used doing something else. How often have you or somebody else said, "I just don't have enough time in the day to get things done?"

A young woman, Ann Makosinski, has never owned a smartphone. She uses a flip phone, and she only got that before she went off to college so that she could keep in touch with her family. Ann grew up without major electronics and had to learn how to entertain herself and make her own toys. She started out making things for herself and then branched out to make things for others.

Her first foray in making things for others was when she found out a friend of hers failed a class in school because she didn't have electricity at home. Ann decided to help her friend, and that's when she came up with a flashlight that is powered by the heat of your hand. She has created other things and has become a very successful young woman, all before the age of 18. She credits her success to not being distracted by the digital world and never having a smartphone. It meant that she had more time in her day to do important things.

Remember those three hours that people spend on their

phones every day? Imagine what you could do during those three hours. What if there was a book that you have wanted to read, but you can't find the time? The average book is around 300 pages. For the average person, this would take around eight hours to read. This time will vary depending on how fast you can read, the book, text size, and content. Now, if you take only an hour out of those three hours, you could read that 300-page book in just over a week.

Maybe you have thought about meditating, but you can't find time to do it. All you have to do is use 30 minutes that you would have otherwise used on your phone.

How's your house looking? Is it a bit cluttered and could use a good cleaning? If you took those three hours you would use on your phone and used them to clean your house; you could clean a three-bedroom house in those three hours.

As you can see, your cell phone use adds up over time. That time could be used to do something more productive, and you could finish things that you have been working on for years.

FOMO and Phubbing

FOMO means the "fear of missing out." This has been used a lot in life, but our smartphones are exacerbating this problem. FOMO is characterized by feeling like you need to know what a person is doing right now and worrying that somebody else is having fun without you. This is why you get so anxious when you hear your phone go off, or when you realize you don't have your phone. You are worried you are going to miss out on something. And that's what leads to phubbing. This FOMO can cause a person to phub a person.

Phubbing is a funny word, but it is a new word used to describe a person who is on their phone while talking to a person in-person. Simply put, it's the phone snubbing. Phubbing was coined in May 2012. It was created by an Australian advertising agency when they noticed a growing phenomenon of people choosing to ignore people right in front of them in favor of scrolling through their phones.

You may have never used the word before, but I'm sure you are familiar with the action. There is a study that found that 17% of people phub others at least four times each day. 32% of people have said that they are phubbed two to three times a day.

While it might not seem like a big, research has found that phubbing can hurt your mental health and your relationships.

Phubbing keeps you from being able to be present in your life and engage with others. A study has found that texting during a regular conversation made that conversation a lot less satisfying for all people involved, even the phubber.

Phubbing and phones can affect marriages as well. It can decrease the satisfaction in a marriage. Conflicts over the spouse's phone use are often the driving force of these issues. It can also increase depression in the spouses.

The effects of phubbing might actually be worse on the person at the receiving end of the phub. There was a study that had participants look at simulated snubbing, and those people felt more negatively about the entire interaction when they were told to picture being the one who is phubbed. What causes these feelings? Phubbing puts are four fundamental needs in danger:

1. Control

2. Meaningful existence

3. Self-esteem

4. Belongingness

When you get phubbed, you feel excluded and rejected. That can have a damaging effect on your mental health. Those people who are phubbed are more likely to use their phones so that they can fill the void.

So how can you know if you are guilty of phubbing?

Here are the three main signs of being a phubber:

1. You hold two conversations at one time, one on your phone and the other in person. You probably aren't having a successful conversation on either end.

2. You immediately start using your phone at dinner or any type of social setting. Sitting your phone right next to your plate "just in case" you get an important message is a major warning sign. Plus, there is no need to touch your phone in order for it to impact the relationship negatively.

3. You never make it through a meal without check your phone. This has to do with FOMO and is a big sign of phubbing.

Phubbing can be stopped, and the following section will discuss five ways to do so. If you notice that somebody is phubbing you, you can always call them out on it. You don't have to be rude or harsh, but let them know that you don't appreciate them using their phone when you are trying to talk to them.

Learning to Control Your Addiction

A third of us will use our phones while we are eating with our friends and families. 50% of people wander around looking down at our phones. 11% of people say that they actually cross the street while using their phones. A third of the population will check their smartphone within five minutes of waking up in the morning. Those are some damning statistics, and those are only some of the statistics.

That said, it's not the device's fault. The fault lies within us and how we use the device. That's actually a good thing, though, because we can control the way we act and use our device. That means we can train ourselves to use our phones responsibly. We are going to go over a few ways in which you can train yourself to stop depending on your phone so much and start paying attention to the world around you.

1. Usage

The first thing you need to understand is your smartphone usage. When you know the reason how you use your smartphone, what you typically use it for, then you can know if you are using it for the right reasons. Moment or Quality Time are apps that you can download that will tell you how you are using your phone. When you get your first analyses of how you use your phone, it will shock you.

Once you can understand the time that is spent using your phone, you can decide if that time is being spent well or not.

2. Living In The Present

This is where you make the conscious decision to focus on those around you. When you are in a social situation, a party, having dinner, shopping, what have you, you put away your phone. Also, ask the people you are with to do the same thing. Turn it off or silence it, and then put it away. Putting somewhere out of sight is very important here. The sight of a phone can reduce our cognitive mental ability. No phone interaction has to occur for this to happen. Merely seeing it can make you dumber.

You have your phone put away, and you will be able to pay attention to others and have a real conversation. You will be able to live in the present.

3. Ask Others to Do The Same

When you are with other people, and they are using their smartphone, just politely ask them to put their smartphone away. The key is to be polite when you do this. Don't demand them, ask them. Explain that you want to give them your full attention, and that would be easier when there aren't any smartphones out.

Your actions of putting your phone away when interacting with people can also be infectious. People will follow your lead if they see you put your phone away first.

4. Don't Sleep with your Phone

A lot of us keep our phones next to our beds at night. By doing this, it makes it more likely that we will gab our phones as soon as we wake up to check what happened overnight. Having the phone in the bedroom can deprive you of sleep. This sleep deprivation can have a mental and physical effect on our wellbeing.

That means you need to find some other place to keep your phone at night. Purchase an alarm clock to wake you up if you need to. You can take this up a level by setting yourself a curfew for when you can use your phone. After that time, turn off your phone and don't use it until the next day.

5. Notifications

Our notifications have created a Pavlov's dog type of

reaction in us. We hear our phone dig, and we start drooling and needing to check it. Notifications increase our inattention and hyperactivity. This all plays into the FOMO that we talked about earlier. We feel like we need to know something right away, but the truth is, it probably isn't all that important.

The best thing to do is just to turn off your notifications. Switch it to airplane mode. This will keep you from being distracted in your life, and you will get more things accomplished.

These five things can help you learn how to function in your life once more. They keep you from being controlled by your phone, and you will then be in control of your phone and life.

Chapter 3: How Your Brain Is Getting Hacked: The Evil Side of Social

Networks

Our gadgets are supposed to make us feel less stressed and more productive, plus they keep us connected to others.

You might have a creeping sensation that they are beginning to do just the opposite. Maybe your significant other is beginning to getting annoyed every tie you pull your smartphone out of your pocket. Maybe you are beginning to sense all that time you take "checking" your social media or email throughout the day is killing the time that you could be doing something else. This includes the larger picture when you think about your life and business.

Anytime you find yourself sucked into your smartphone or become distracted, you may think it's all because of you or maybe an accident that you picked your phone up again. But it isn't. It is because the apps on smartphones can hijack our natural psychological vulnerabilities and biases.

How can you know if you are truly addicted to your phone? If you do realize that you should cut back, how will you be able to manage your technology addiction in check? You are an entrepreneur, and you aren't going to throw your cell phone away and move to a cabin in the woods.

I figured out about the minds' vulnerabilities when I worked as a magician. They have to look for biases, openness, and blind spots in a person's mind so that they can influence what all of their users do without realizing it. Once you figure out how to push other people's buttons, you can play them. Technology ends up doing this with our minds. App designers use the vulnerabilities to grab a person's attention.

Your Cell Phone Is a Slot Machine

If you are an app, how can you keep people coming back? Simple, it becomes a slot machine.

Each day, the average person will check their phone about 150 times. Why? Are those 150 choices conscious? The main reason why a slot machine is so addictive is that it uses intermittent variable rewards.

If you want something to be as addictive as possible, tech designers have to reward the actions of the user in some way. The user's efforts in this scenario are pulling the lever on a slot machine. You pull that lever, and you immediately get either nothing or an enticing reward like a prize or match. Your addiction gets maximized when you don't know what to expect.

Does this actually work on people? Absolutely, slot machines bring in more money than theme parks, movies, and baseball combined in a year's time as related to different types of gambling because a person can become addicted to a slot machine about four times faster.

Makes You Feel Like You Belong

Here is the bad news, but it is also the truth: Billions of

people keep a tiny form of a slot machine in their pocket.

After it gets pulls out of your pocket, you are playing the slots to see if you have received any notifications. Once you swipe to begin scrolling through your Instagram feed, you are playing the slots to see what picture pops up next. Anytime you refresh your email, you are playing the slots to see what message you received. Then you move on to Tinder to see if you can find a match. You begin swiping faces, and again you are playing the slots.

There are times when this happens intentionally because websites and apps throw in variable rewards throughout their products because they know they can suck you into their web this way. At other times like when you are checking your phone or email, it is purely accidental.

One more way technology kidnaps your mind is by inducing a one percent chance that you might be missing out on essential things. Apps will also exploit the fact that we all seek approval. Anytime you see a notification that says: "Your friend Sam tagged you in…" you feel like you have been instantly approved by your friend, and you feel like you belong. Tech companies are at the center of all of this.

Snapchat, Instagram, or Facebook manipulates the number of times a person gets tagged by suggesting faces for us to tag. When a friend tags you, they are actually responding to a suggestion from Facebook. At this point, you aren't making independent choices. With design choices like these, Facebook can control how often millions, if not billions of people, can experience social approval.

This occurs whenever you change your profile picture. Facebook understands that at that moment, you are the most vulnerable to social approval because you are wondering what your friends will think about your new picture. Facebook will end up placing this higher in the newsfeed so that it sticks around and more people see and comments on it. Each time that happens, you get sucked back in.

Everybody naturally responds to approval on social media, but demographics for teenagers are a lot more vulnerable than others. This is why it is important to notice all the power designers hold when they choose to use this vulnerability.

An Empire

LinkedIn wants people to create social obligations for one another as often as possible. Every time one of them reciprocates by endorsing somebody or responding to messages, they have to go back to the app where they suck people into spending more time there.

Just like Facebook, LinkedIn uses a lack of equality in perception. If somebody sends you an invite to connect with them, you think they made a conscious decision to invite you, but they really just responded to a suggested contact on LinkedIn. Basically, LinkedIn causes your impulses to become obligations so that people feel like they have to reciprocate. Meanwhile, LinkedIn is profiting from all the time that people are spending on their website.

Welcome to the social media empire. Western culture has been built on the ideals of freedom and individual choice. People will always fight for our rights to get to make our own choices, but the one thing that we all ignore is how our options get manipulated by menus that we didn't get to pick out.

This is what magicians do. People think they have been given a choice while creating the menu, so they ultimately win, and it won't matter what you pick.

If a person is given numerous choices, they aren't going to ask: "What's not on the menu?" "Why do I have to make a choice and not others?" "Do I know what they want?" "Is this going to help me out, or distract me?"

Let's say it's Thursday night, and you are out with your friends, and you would like the conversation to continue. You open up your Yelp App to find some nearby bars. Then, magically, the group becomes a bunch of people staring at their phones comparing bars. They closely look at every photo and begin comparing drinks. Is this even relevant to what the group wanted?

What If You Aren't Hungry?

I'm not saying that going to bars isn't a good choice. It is just Yelp substituted the original question of "where can we go to keep talking?" with the question, "Which one has better photos?" The bad this is, the friends fell for this idea that the Yelp menu provides them with a different group of choices.

When technology provides us with a choice in several areas of our lives, the more we start to think that our phones are useful to choose from. Is this the truth? If you stopped to ask yourself, "Who isn't attached that I can go out with," you will quickly find yourself swiping through thousands of faces on Tinder instead of going someplace that you and your friends can enjoy. "Who doesn't have any plans," turns into a menu of people you send out texts to. "What's going on," gives you a newsfeed of the lasting happenings.

Businesses maximized all their "time spent" design within apps to make us consume more things, even if we aren't hungry. How do they do this? They have turned something that was finite and bounded into a bottomless pit of pointless information that never comes to an end.

Brian Wansink, a professor at Cornell, showed how this could happen by showing how people can be tricked into continuing to eat soup when the bowls are bottomless. The bowl would automatically refill every time the person eats some of the soup. People will eat about 73 percent more soup with bottomless bowls than normal bowls.

This is the same principle used by tech companies. Our newsfeeds are made to automatically refill with new information that makes you want to continue to scroll. They purposely remove anything that could make your pause, leave, or reconsider.

This is why social and video media platforms like Facebook, YouTube, and Netflix will automatically play the very next show after about a 15-second countdown rather than giving you the chance to decide if you want to continue watching.

Common Tragedies

Tech companies like to claim they are just trying to make their user's lives easier. They think they are catering to their users' best interests. You can't really blame them since increasing the time spent on their website is the money they compete for.

Companies know that interruptions are great for their business, too. Suppose given a choice, Facebook Messenger, Snapchat, or WhatsApp like to make their systems to interrupt a person right away rather than giving users the chance to respect each other's attention since their response is more likely to be immediate. It's better for them if they make it feel more urgent. Facebook will automatically tell the sender if you saw the message, rather than allowing you to avoid disclosing that you read it or not. Because of this, you feel as if you have to respond.

The issue of maximizing the interruptions just to create more business will create what is called the tragedy of the commons. This ruins the global attention span and causes billions of interruptions daily that could have been avoided.

Does it upset you knowing that your technology hijacks your actions? Me, too. I have only listed some of the techniques they use, but there are thousands more. Think about training, workshops, seminars, and bookshelves that teach all those aspiring young techies all these techniques. Visualize rooms full of engineers whose job is to create new ways to keep you addicted to their app.

This wasn't written to make you depressed, or to make you think you have to give up your phone. This isn't a one-or-nothing approach. Do we want to live in a world where we can't use our cell phones or use them and get hijacked constantly?

Billions of people inevitably have a phone in their

pocket, but they could be made to do something other than making us addicted to them. You have the chance to demand that the tech world provides us with something different. This is similar to the time everyone demanded to have better food, and the organic food movement began.

"Time Well Spent" Internet

Rather than maximizing a user's "time spent," think about what it would be like if apps offered an alternate, paid, or hybrid types of services that could maximize "time well spent," and they gave them a special rank within search engines and the app store. Visualize if you will rather than releasing new phones every year, Google and Apple created phones to protect the user's from becoming addicted but will empower them to make their own choices. Just think about if we have a "digital bill of rights" that specifies a standard for all websites and apps to follow. For example, the design would force the app to give the user one way to find what they want rather than what the app wants you to do. Think about what would happen if companies had to get rid of or reduce the slot machine effect by changing up the variable reward into something that is predictable and less addictive. They could give the user the power to set specific times during their week or day for checking the "slot machine" apps and being able to change how new messages get delivered.

Think about what it would be like if these companies would help us shape our relationships, business, and friends in ways of what we think is "time well spent" for us rather than in what we think we will be missing. Visualize an organization that is interested in the interests of the public that helped to define specific standards and then watched for when the companies abused these standards.

Think about smartphones and web browsers and the way people make choices. What if the companies behind that technology watched out for their users and helped them know how every click could affect them. If you tell a person the truth about what a click could cost them, you are treating them with respect and dignity. Within a "time well spent" internet, choices are going to get framed in terms of benefit and possible cost to make sure that people can make the best choice available to them without having to do any more work.

"Ultimate freedom is a free mind," we need to have technology that works for us, so we can act freely, think, feel, and live.

We need smartphones to be the interpersonal relationships and exoskeletons of our minds that put values first. Let us protect our minds with as much strictness as privacy and all the other digital rights.

Likes Are The New Nicotine

It has been said that "social media is the new smoking, and it's an addiction." You know what? I believe them. Social media is very much a double-edged sword. It can do a lot for people, especially small businesses. It can help bring in customers, improve networking, and help people connect with others. But it is also hazardous, as we have discussed already.

What's more, is the developer of the "endless scroll" has come forward recently and apologized for the impact that it has had on society. But let's back up to the smoking analogy. Social media started life a lot as smoking did.

When smoking made its breakout into the mass marketplace, it sold like hotcakes. People couldn't get enough of lighting up, and everybody "tried" smoking in some way, shape, or form. Puffing straights, rolling your own, whatever your smoked, you were considered cool. Over time, though, specifically at the turn of the Century, as more research was being conducted on smoking, doctors and scientists discovered that smoke was very bad.

While most people believe that smokers came from smoking families, kids who had parents who never smoked still chose to try cigarettes. The reason they did this was because of popularity. They want to fit in.

Their friends try it, so they do as well. It's part of the developmental process of the human mind, and it's completely normal. That doesn't mean everybody will try smoking, but there will be something they try just because their friends do.

The CEO of Salesforce, Marc Benioff, has stated that social media addiction is like smoking by explaining that companies like Facebook need to be regulated "exactly the same way you've made the cigarette industry accountable," by putting consumer safety before the companies money.

But how can we liken social media to smoking, which is very much a deadly habit? Let's look at some facts.

Mark Zuckerberg, in a *New Yorker* article, described Facebook's business as such, "This is an inherently cultural thing. It's at the intersection of technology and psychology, and it's very personal." Facebook's employees don't have a degree in psychology, and they definitely aren't trying to help people, yet the tactics that the company uses are created in a way that is meant to trigger psychological responses in us.

A few years ago, Facebook began to experiment with people's newsfeeds to see if negative news caused people to act more pessimistic online, and if positive posts would help them be kind. They did not disclose what they were doing, nor did they ask for permission from the users. They worked around this because of the terms of service that everybody had to agree to before they made their account.

It's not just Facebook, though. Every form of social media is addictive in some way. Maximizing engagement is what they are all about. The more time that you spend clicking and scrolling through their app, the better it is for their business.

What's worse is that studies have found that social media is more addictive than cigarettes. They say that the allure of Twitter or Facebook is harder to resist than the urge to light up after a big meal.

Within the studies about the addiction of social media, they found that most social media platforms have a negative effect on a person's wellbeing with an exception. YouTube actually has an overall positive impact on a person's well-being. Instagram has the worst effect on a person's mental health.

Let's all take a moment and think about our grandparents. None of them had a mobile phone when growing up. There's a chance that they didn't even have a landline, and if they did, it was definitely a party line. They didn't message people on Facebook. Instead, they had to physically meet up in person, at a set time and place. They interacted with people. I'm not saying the past was better than the present. I'm very grateful for the things we have, but they had something that the younger generation may not learn about if they don't put down their phone.

Whenever you take a pug off of that cigarette, or you get a "like" on your photo, you are hit with dopamine. It is this good feeling that makes you keep coming back and wanting more. Younger people love it when they get this buzz of "positive" energy, and they simply can't get enough of it. A single cigarette every few hours will turn into one every few minutes. A single post every few days turns into a post every hour. You end up becoming dependent and then addicted.

When the Wi-Fi goes out, or you don't have the money to buy another pack, the dopamine dependant person stops, and then crashes. This crash leaves them feeling like they can't function, and it causes bad moods, low self-esteem, and then bad mental health.

With each new generation, young people are getting more access to smartphones and other devices. This is making the physical effects of social media more prevalent in society.

Social Networks Manipulate Your Brain

Is there a way you can live your life staying away from the manipulations and distractions of other people? In order to do this, you have to know the way you work. You have to "know thyself," as the ancients have urged us to do. Most of the time, we are very bad at this.

In contrast, other people have a very good understanding of who we are. They know who we like, our intelligence, and anything else that can be computed from our likes on Facebook. The machines that use this data from what we look at on our devices know our personality better than our family and friends. It won't be long before this type of artificial intelligence knows a lot more about us. Our challenge is knowing the best way to live when others already know so much about us.

Are we really free today? Many companies are dedicated to capturing and then selling what we pay attention to; their best bait is social media. Twitter, Instagram, and Facebook have brought many people closer together. But these do come with a cost both political and personal. Users have to decide if all the benefits they get from these apps and websites are worth what they cost them.

You have to make this decision freely. Can we be free if social media sites are addictive? This is another decision that should be an informed one. Could it be that we have no clue as to who is behind the curtain?

Facebook's first president, Sean Parker, had talked about the process that was used when they came up with the site. Parked explained that, "All about how do we consume as much of your time and conscious attention as possible?"

To reach this goal, they need to make sure that the user got, "A little dopamine hit every once in a while because someone liked or commented on a photo or a post, and that's going to get you to contribute more."

He continued with, "It's exactly the kind of thing that a hacker like myself would come up with because you're exploiting a vulnerability in human psychology... the inventors, creators, it's me, it's Mark... understood this consciously. And we did it anyway."

Our Needs Create Our Vulnerabilities

What are the vulnerabilities of humans? We all have this need to belong, and we want to achieve meaningful social status. Because of this, the brain will treat whatever information we find on ourselves as something special, a reward. If we get our behaviors rewarded through things like money or food, our brains have a "valuation system" that gets activated. Most of this system can be started if we find relevant information about ourselves. Our minds give this information a lot of weight. This is why, when you hear somebody call your name from across the room, it is going to appear in your consciousness.

We feel that any type of information that is connected to our social rank and reputation is crucial. We are all wired to be sensitive towards these types of things. Social dominance is understood by the time we are 15 months old.

Social media sites grab hold of us because they involve information that is relevant to ourselves, and they bear our reputation and social status. This makes you want to be popular and belong even more, and the more our brain's reward center responds to the enhancement of our reputation, the more we hear the "siren's song" of the media site.

Every time you log into Twitter, Facebook, Google, or any other "free" social media sites, all the information from each keystroke gets fed into a powerful computer somewhere. These computers use algorithms to correlate this data. They then compare you to others who have profiles that are similar to yours. These algorithms are intelligent but blind. They do various experiments to use information in different ways to see if it can change your actions so that you do what they want you to do. They want their users to respond to ads for a certain service or product. They can be trying to convince you to vote a certain way.

An entrepreneur and scientist, Jaron Lanier, pioneered virtual reality. He talks about the questionable use of the personal data collected by social media networks. He isn't trying to use his book to get people to leave social media altogether. Still, he wants to warn you against all the harmful side effects of social media like mind manipulation and addiction. Lanier gives suggestions about how social media can be changed.

The large digital companies make use of algorithms to find more information about you that you didn't actually share. They want to figure out how to attract and hold your attention so paid clients, politicians, and advertisers can influence you for their purposes. The data that they collect includes facial expressions, the way in which you move your body, the people you are friends with, your favorite books, where you go, what you eat, and how easily you are to persuade. They then use this data to create stimulus feeds that can be either unpaid or paid that are designed to increase your "engagement" and increase how effective their advertisement was. The executives have Facebook have admitted that they used all of these addictive qualities deliberately. This is why it should be called "behavior modification stimuli" or addiction.

Advertising has changed a lot from the print variety to digital. When advertising we available only in print, it was a one-way relationship. The advertiser would send out an ad and hoped they would get some customers. Within the world of digital media, advertising comes with connections that people already have. How ads work on social platforms involves the monitoring of the users so that they know what is in the ad so they can personalize the stream until the user's behavior gets changed. Some forms of stimuli can influence almost every social media user.

Positive stimuli could include retweets, friending, or helping a video go viral. Negative stimuli might consist of any occurrence of being unappreciated, ridiculed, or unnoticed. The bad news is that both negative and positive emotions have power over us, but they are timed differently. Positive emotions take a longer time to build up, and if not sustained, can easily be lost. Negative emotions happen faster, but they go away a lot slower. It takes a lot longer to gain a person's trust than it takes to lose their trust. A person could get angry or afraid quickly, but it will take a long time for those feelings to go away. The bad consequences that nobody realized is that all those negative emotions are more emphasized since positive ones take a long time to show up, and this can influence the way paying customers use social media to manipulate society and normal users.

One other problem with social media is that it is a huge gateway for news. This means that more people are going to be getting news that pushes their buttons. It can't be anything else because this material is created by people who aren't who they pretend to be. It can also be created by computers and distributed by robots.

Social media can be used to bring people together, but conspiracy theories, xenophobia, paranoia, and anger create more engagement. Social media will show you things that stimulate emotions that were listed earlier because it is easier to create feelings of fear, resentment, and anger than emotions of security, affection, and joy. This can corrupt politics very quickly. Feedback on social media is meant to reinforce whatever your feelings are, whether it is anti-war, pro-gun, conservative, or liberal, and this keeps you from being able to understand others who don't think the same way you do. Social media can increase all the divisions in society.

Social media actually operates below people's awareness levels. The best way you can find out just how much you have been influenced is to switch off your accounts for a six month period and see how things go. This is going to show you just how much social media had been affecting you and if it would be worth your time to continue using them. Do you think a large number of people will do this? At one time, there was a large number of people who no one thought would stop smoking actually stopped. The main problem is social media that is based on advertising.

To me, this problem is a lot deeper. I think it is within the nature of technology and the economy. Traditional media have used the majority of social media's tricks. During the 90s, newspapers tried to find out which type of news the readers wanted. They did focus groups and surveys, and they saw most people wanted positive news. When asked what article they could remember the best, the response was the article on the baby that was found dead in a dumpster. This didn't mean that the people were hypocrites. Humans tend to react in ways that we don't pick; this is what causes us to get manipulated.

Some people might argue that Netflix and Amazon use the same algorithms to suggest videos and books that you might be interested in, but this is done with the intention of getting business from you and not to influence you to benefit a third party. The main problem is Google and Facebook's business model. These have been created to grab your attention, and then they sell that to third parties. Regulation is going to fix this. If profit is what is motivating them, then they are going to find a way around the rules. The best way to fix this issue would be through a brand new set of business models where social media sites earn money off of their users instead of third parties. The benefits from this would be social media users are the customer and not a product. This solution involves charging people to use their service, and this suggests that charges would be affordable for most people. The payments can be made in pennies or a fraction of cents.

Social media does use a lot of manipulation, but implementing the suggestions above would be extremely hard to do. Newspapers, when they were powerful and influential, weren't every able to be free from depending on advertisers. Most profitable newspapers or other print publications are complementary, and they make their profits from the income they get from their advertisers. Some don't use advertisers and have to depend on subscriptions. They also rely on donations to help make ends meet. The economics of social media is a lot different from newspapers, and maybe some of the suggestions above might be feasible. There is the issue of getting a business that is profitable without any competitors to give up what makes them money.

How to Take Control

How can you benefit from social platforms without getting addicted to them? Companies have the option of changing their sites to diminish addiction risk. They could decide to use an opt-out setting for features that strengthen addictions. This will make it easier for people to regulate how much they use the site. Some companies claim that asking these technology companies "to be less good at what they do feels like a ridiculous ask." We might need to get some help from the government like we did to fight the tobacco industry.

Users can also assess their personal reasons that could be causing them to be more vulnerable to problem usage. Some things that could cause excessive use might include a bigger tendency to have a fear of missing out, feeling lonely, needed self-promotion, not being able to cope with daily problems, and experiencing negative emotions. These factors aren't going to apply to all people.

Users could also empower themselves. You can limit the time you spend on these sites by using other apps like StayFocused, Moment, and Freedom. Most Facebook users have taken breaks from Facebook voluntarily, but this is hard for some.

To quote the most famous line from *Invictus*: "I am the master of my fate, I am the captain of my soul." Future generations might find this incomprehensible.

It's All Engineered

All of this addiction to social media does not happen by accident. It is all engineered by the gurus in Silicon Valley. They planned everything out, and they wanted it to be had for us to say no. I mentioned the creator of the infinite scroll in an earlier chapter, well, Aza Raskin also had this to say, "it's as if they're taking behavioral cocaine and just sprinkling it all over your interface. And that's the thing that keeps you coming back and back and back." The infinite scroll makes users of Facebook, Instagram, and Tiktok stay longer on the platform.

Tech insiders in Silicon Valley have started to speak up about these products and what they are doing to us. Chamath Palihapitiya, a former vice president for Facebook, said, "I feel tremendous guilt... I think we have created tools that are ripping apart the social fabric of how society works."

With everything you see on your phone, there have been thousands of engineers coming up with ways to maximize the addictive nature of the app. The platforms will test how to lure users back, from how the like button is shaped to the sounds and colors they use.

Sean Parker, the first president of Facebook, explained that Facebook is becoming "a social-validation feedback look." Our behaviors, identity, and beliefs are shaped by the interactions we have with other people. This includes people we have known for a long time and just fleeting moments of eye contact with a stranger. Past generations had a respite from this social world, but with social media and smartphones have given us access to this contact a lot easier.

All of this constant influx of information has an effect on us. Despite the saying that nothing on the internet goes away, social information can become less meaningful and expire with time, for example, direct messages, live streams, and ongoing groups. When people don't keep up with them, that's when people start experiencing FOMO. That's the thing, though, the creators of all of your favorite social platforms want this to happen.

We all know FOMO happens when we are disconnected, such as losing signal or having a dead battery, but that FOMO happens while we are connected. For example, if a person has multiple devices and social accounts and doesn't have the time or desire to check all of them, they can start worrying about missing important events and messages.

FOMO can also show up when people get frustrated that others haven't responded, even though they have received and read the message. There are other subcategories to this that the engineers play into as well, such as:

- Fear of inciting negative reactions.

- Fear of not being included in a social group due to a lack of timely engagement.

- Fear of missing important information.

- Fear of missing the chance to gain popularity.

The design features of the apps trigger these responses in their users. For example, letting us know the number of likes that a person's post receives can cause fear in another that they are missing out on approval. WhatsApp has a double tick delivery and notification feature, and this can create a preoccupation with social relationships. The streak feature on Snapchat, which keeps track of the number of days in a row that you spent using the app, and makes users feel like they need to check in with the app each day to keep up their streak.

Notifications are a completely different beast. In a lot of messaging apps, there is a mark that shows when they have read the message. Both parties are a way of those tick marks, so that creates social pressure to respond. Sometimes you get sent an email that tells you that you have a new message, which just adds more stress, lest you were to miss out on something important. And then you have those horrible bubbles that show up when a person is typing in a reply. What are the odds that you are going to put down that phone before they send you a response?

You may still be wondering why they would do something like this. It's important to remember that for those social media companies, the main objective is to make money. Facebook is worth $835.27B as of August 2020, but anybody who has an account can tell you that it doesn't cost to have an account. While this may seem contradictory, it isn't. We can use Facebook for free because we aren't their real customers. Their advertisers a the real customers, and they sell our attention. Look at it this way, the more often you are on social media, the more chance you have to see an ad. Every minute spends on Facebook is another minute spent helping make money for somebody else.

It also gives them another minute to collect data from you that they can sell to others. Facebook is a huge collector of personal data. Facebook has also shared "success stories" of how companies have used their abilities to slice, analyze, and predict things using the data to target certain customers.

Regardless of how you feel about this type of data collection, it explains the reasons why social media companies want to make sure that you continue to come back and continue to use the app for a long time. This is how they make their money. They have to make sure their app manipulates us to achieve this goal. This is where our slot machine analogy comes into play.

We've said it time and time again; the infinite scroll is a big player in keeping people hooked. The companies have removed any type of cues that could stop our scrolling, such as come to the bottom of a page, which gives you a moment to decide to do something different. The ethical video game creators have started to add cues to help break up their games into chapters. This gives the players a chance to play their game in small chunks without facing long binges. Instagram, Facebook, and Twitter do not use that. They are the bottomless pits of the social world. If there was a natural end, it would help their users to move onto something else.

We have what is called a ventral tegmental area (VTA). This is the main area that is responsible for determining the rewards system in our body. When a user receives a like or positive feedback, the brain will fire off dopamine receptors, which is control, partly, but the VTA. Even MRIs of the brain during social media users have found similar results.

We have mentioned this dopamine response several times, but let's take a moment to look at why we have this dopamine response, to begin with. From an evolutionary standpoint, dopamine was released in response to having sex or eating. But our dopamine system isn't able to tell the difference between a habit that helps and a habit that harms. Dopamine reinforces our habits, even those that are bad, and that's how we get addicted to things.

There is no denying the fact their these features are effective, but while it is great for their business, it isn't all that great for our mental health. As long as they continue to profit off of selling our attention, nothing is going to change in how they do things. Short of government intervention or pressure from their consumers, it is pretty hard to imagine that these companies are going to get rid of their hooks and mark their products safer for our mental health.

Thankfully, though, there are ways that we can take our mental health into our own hands. Sure, it's going to hurt their businesses because they aren't getting our attention, but they will make money elsewhere. We have to make sure that we look out for ourselves and make sure we escape from their traps and hooks. It's also important that we teach our children about this as well. Facebook, and other social networks, target the younger demographics so that they are trapped early on. It's our job to make sure that this doesn't happen. You'll be happy that you did.

Chapter 4: How They

Manipulate Your Brain: The Vegas Effect and Desire for Social Approval

At this point, we have a very good understanding as to why social media and the digital world is so addictive. The people who create those apps and all of the content creates in with psychological mechanisms in mind to attract people and to keep them there. We've said that likes are the new nicotine and that social media is like a slot machine. To that end, they also use what is known as the Vegas effect, along with an intermittent reinforcement schedule and our need to feel approved by our friends. They hit us where we are the weakest, and they exploit those weaknesses.

In 2018, there were 2.5 billion smartphones in use around the world. There are about 7.7 billion people on the planet, so that's a lot of smartphones. Then you have social media. Snapchat has around 200 million users. Instagram has around 400 million users. Facebook has over 2.25 billion users. That means almost everybody who has a smartphone also has a Facebook account. We've already figured out that Facebook is one of the worst social media platforms to use.

Let's focus on just America for a moment. The average American will spend 1460 hours each year on their smartphone. If we assume that people sleep eight hours each night, that means we spend 91 waking days each year on our phones. But they do have an extraordinary power over us that makes it very hard to put our phone down and do something else.

Vegas Effect and Intermittent Reinforcement Schedules

There are various reasons why it is hard to put our phones down. This includes supernormal stimuli and classical conditioning. There is another mechanism that hooks us into continually checking our phones for the latest information. This is also why people are drawn to "loot boxes" in video games. This is what is known as a variable ratio reinforcement schedule.

B.F. Skinner was a behaviorist and psychologist who studied how people responded to certain things and how it was established and strengthened through schedules of reinforcement. For example, a pigeon placed in a box learns that if he pecks at a bar, he gets a food pellet, and then learns that he only gets the pellet for every three pecks of the lever. This is a type of fixed-interval reinforcement schedule. Any kind of reinforcement schedule is created through operant conditioning.

This is a learning process where new behavior is

acquired and modified through an association with a consequence. When you reinforce an action, there is a better chance that it is going to happen again, while punishing a behavior lowers the chance that it is going to happen again. This plays a part in punishing or rewarding a child for their actions.

These reinforcement schedules can happen in natural learning situations and in structured training situations. In the real-world, behaviors are not likely to get reinforced each time they happen. In situations where people want to intentionally reinforce a certain action, like animal training, sports, or school, they would use a specific reinforcement schedule. Some schedules work better for certain situations. Some training may need one schedule, and the change to another once a certain behavior has been achieved.

We have two foundational forms of reinforcement schedules, partial and continuous. With continuous reinforcement, the behavior gets reinforced every time it happens. This is what most people will use during the initial stages of learning so that there is a strong connection between response and behavior. For example, if you want to teach your dog to shake hands, during the first stages of learning, you would continuously reinforce so that they can establish the behavior. This would involve taking the dog's paw whenever you say shake. Then you reward the dog every time you do this. Eventually, the dog will begin to do the action whenever you say shake.

After the response has been established, you would switch to a partial reinforcement schedule. This is when the behavior gets reinforced part of the time. The learned actions get acquired at a slower rate. With the dog training, you will eventually move to a partial schedule to provide more reinforcement after the behavior is established. There are four types of partial reinforcement.

First, you have a fixed-ratio schedule. You reinforce the action after a specific number of times. This will create a high, steady rate of response with a brief pause from the reinforcement.

Second is a variable-ratio schedule. This happens when

81

behavior gets reinforced after an unpredictable amount of responses. This will cause a high, steady rate of responses. The lottery and gambling are examples of this type of schedule.

The third is the fixed-interval schedule. This is where the first response is rewarded only after a certain amount of time has passed. This causes a high amount of answers close to the end of the interval, but a slower response immediately after delivery by the reinforce.

Fourth is the variable-interval schedules. This is where the reward happens at an unpredictable amount of time after the response occurs. This causes a slow and steady rate of reaction.

The one that affects the way we use our phones is a variable ratio reinforcement schedule, so let's take a look at that.

You get a variable ratio reinforcement when, after a certain number of actions, some type of reward is achieved. With the pigeon example, the pigeon doesn't know how many times he has to peck the lever to get the food. One time he just pecks it once, and other times he has to do it five times, or 20. The research will randomize the distribution so that the pigeon will never figure out how many pecks will give him the food. It figures out that the more often he pecks at the lever, the sooner he will likely get food.

Researchers have discovered that these types of schedules often result in a high rate of response. Also, these variable ratios are resistant to extinction. With the pigeon, even if the researcher were to stop giving the birds food, the pigeon is still going to peck at the lever and for a long time until it gives up. Slot machines, and any other games of chance, are perfect examples of this variable ratio schedule.

As it turns out, the variable schedule tends to be involved in a lot of behavioral addictions, like gambling. That means, in a sense, compulsively eyeing your phone is like compulsive gambling. This is what is known as the "Vegas effect." This means that we can experience an almost feverish compulsion to engage in certain actions. In fact, there are plenty of "obsessions" and hobbies that use this variable reinforcement, like:

- Hunting

- Fishing

- Channel surfing

- Looking for bargains while shopping

- Any type of collecting

Why is this type of reinforcement so powerful? This variable, or intermittent, reinforcement is unpredictable random rewards that happen after repeated behavior. Still, there is a powerful formula at play that makes a person feel the need to act in this way. This need can be elevated gradually and subtly to extreme levels, which creates compliance that can be obsessive and sometimes self-destructive. The more infrequently the food pellets of love are offered, the more hooked we become.

Variable reinforcement isn't a bad thing on its own. They play a very important part in motivation and the learning system in the brain. This is how we end up learning about casual relationships. When you look at it from an evolutionary standpoint, learning causal relationships improves our chances of survival. For example, if I do this, then it's important that I learn if this particular outcome is likely to happen. When we discover that there is a variable relationship, we know that if we do A, we might get B. Our reward system will then release dopamine in these variable situations to help motivate us to pay attention so we can learn about this connection. This is also known as incentive salience. Basically, the brain motives us to "crack the code."

More importantly, is that this dopamine reward system often involves wanting versus liking. We get a rush of dopamine more often when we anticipate that something might occur. For example, if little Jimmy purchases a pack of baseball cards and is getting ready to open, he will experience a release of dopamine before he actually opens the pack. This means that the dopamine is incentivizing little Jimmy to open the pack, as well as purchasing more.

Lab rats learn to press lever by giving them a continuous positive reinforcement. That means, to start out with, each time they press a lever, they are given a morsel of food. Then the research will change it up. The rat will press the lever for food but doesn't get anything. He starts getting worried that he won't be fed again, but he knows that the lever gave him food before, so he continuously presses the lever until he receives food. As long as the researcher still gives him some food every once and a while, the rate will continue to press the lever to make sure he gets food.

This is the same way that traumatic bonding happens. A trauma bond is simply a strong attachment to an abuser that gets developed not in spite of the abuse, but because of it.

This intermittent reinforcement starts out insidiously and will escalate at a gradual pace. We get our first phone and start texting our friends. The messages come regularly, but then, slowly, they come when we don't expect them. You could even find yourself stewing over the fact that your friend hasn't messaged you back in a day or two, even though you know they have read the message. You're ready to throw in the towel on your friendship when you finally get a reply. All of that anger is forgotten, and then you start pecking at that lever once more.

It is relatively easy to see how technology, like gaming, texting, and social media, works using a variable reinforcement schedule. Just like a box of chocolate, we don't know what we are going to get. Who shared a post on Facebook? Who commented on my update? I have to check my email. My phone just buzzed, and wondered what it was about? I just need to check the news feed one more time.

As soon as our phones buzz, it activates this dopamine reward system. Again, it is this anticipation that will activate our reward system. We have to find out what happened, no matter what it is. It's like a bug bite that's itching, and you just have to scratch it. It's like the pigeon pecking at the lever in the hopes that it will receive food. We continue to check out phones. As much as all of us want to believe that we are above getting addicted to these types of compulsive behaviors, we often behave like a pigeon in a box. It's also important to understand that this reinforcement schedule does not just happen with technology or the like; it can also occur in relationships.

Our Need for Approval

We're going take a little detour here and talk about the human nature of needing approval. We'll bring this back around to our phones and the digital world in a moment.

When our relationships start getting messy, we will end the relationship, but there are some who struggle with letting go. Why? Metaphorically, who likes to be shut out of a locked house? We all long to be able to open that closed door.

We've all faced this problem in one way or another. It's hard to lose a relationship, and it is even harder to come to terms with accepting what we can't control. Those doors get closed for a reason, yet it still hurts, but why does it hurt?

The reason it hurts so much is our need for approval. The humanistic psychologist, Abraham Maslow, placed belongingness within our hierarchy of needs but also argued that it is a necessity. Seeking approval means you seek acceptance. It is your sense of belonging. These are all fundamental aspects of our emotional development and wellbeing. When we feel like others approve of us, we have more self-assurance and self-esteem. These are emotions that help us thrive because they motivate us, help us move forward, and survive. That means seeking approval is something that we do instinctually.

Children are taught early on to seek approval from their parents for what they say or do. Since this is a strong connection with our parents, we become conditioned, over time, to seek the approval of others. When we don't get approval from a person, it triggers a need to win it back. When we don't receive approval, we don't feel protected and safe.

Look at it this way, how often do your run most of your decisions past people in your life, like family members, friends, therapist, or people on your social media? Probably more often than you want to admit. You do this because you need approval. You want to make sure people already like what you are going to do before you ever do it. This need to seek approval can affect your relationships and career because you are always worried about what others will think.

It's one thing for teens to measure their worth through the number of likes they get, they are still mentally developing, but when it's somebody who should know better, it looks desperate.

This isn't a straight forward process. To seek approval means you have to find approval. As stated earlier, we are greatly impacted early on in our development through expectations and experiences. Carl Rogers explains this by saying, "molds who we are to who we should be." Nevertheless, this need to belong doesn't end when we grow older. All you need to look at is the fact that we are willing to change things about ourselves in order to get the validation and approval that we are seeking. This is what makes Instagram so dangerous to our self-esteem.

With social media, this is why so many people lose their authenticity or their true-selves. People are willing to do whatever they have to in order to be cool. This is all due to an instinctual drive to be approved by others and meet a deep-rooted need to belong. But, how far is a person willing to go to feel like they belong?

To get an idea of how far humans are willing to go, let's take a look at something that happened in 2016. A 24-year-old Canadian woman, Melina Roberge, started smuggling cocaine on cruise liners, where she would then take selfies and photos. Her reason for doing this was "governed by a superficial desire to take pictures of myself in exotics locations to post on Instagram and receive likes and attention." This choice would end up sending her to jail.

This is a part of the external validation problem many

people have. Basically, they seek the approval of others in order to feel worthy of themselves. Insecure people, and those with fragile egos, are more susceptible to seek out external opinions to feel good about themselves.

A narcissist falls within this. At a subclinical level, these people will have traits that include acting entitled, superior, and behaving in a grandiose manner. To go so far as to say Melina is a narcissist is making the jump. However, her need for attention from her followers does make one wonder about her self-esteem. This is something that everybody needs to think about when they feel compelled to judge others in similar situations.

It's important to understand that a person's confidence or self-esteem is not the same thing as narcissism. There are those who are extremely confident. They get unfairly labeled as a narcissist. The thing is, there is a big difference between those two types of people. While narcissists are people you likely want to avoid; the confident person is the type of person you can count on for guidance. You might like to know how to spot the difference. It's actually not all that difficult.

Narcissists choose dominance. People who are confident favor equality. Narcissists have qualities like denigration, arrogance, and criticism. Confident people have qualities like respect, constructive feedback, and humility. This can be explained by the fact that those who have a healthy about of self-esteem have built their confidence through moral values, real achievements, and they care and respect others. This isn't how it works for the narcissist. Their actions are completely fuelled by the fear of failure, insecurity, and inadequacy. You can easily see how social media can help to get rid of those types of feelings. It gives a person the chance to build up a sense of belonging and find validation through a simple thumbs-up, but that's kind of dangerous.

The person-centered approach of Carl Rogers presents the idea of the flexible self. However, it talks about the idea that people can only distance themselves from who they truly are up to a certain point. Once they reach that point, they enter the stage of incongruence, which explains what causes human emotional distress, and conflict. It is the grey area of the psyche where things become unrecognizable, including ourselves.

The flexibility of the self gives us the chance to explore new territories, recreate, and rediscover who we are. This is an important part of life, as it helps us to mature, psychologically grow, and change horizons. For this to occur, however, we have to know who we are. Why? To make sure we don't betray our core values and forgetting what drives us. This will allow you to negotiate and find a balance between your inner requirements and those of society. This will make you able to feel genuine acceptance, belonging, and love. This will lead to a life of healthy self-assurance and self-esteem. This is a state that makes it possible for us not only to receive appreciation and love but to return those things to communities and individuals.

There is one social media maven who has seen the problem with social media. Essena O'Neill, from Australia, announced that she would be going to give up social media because it was making her "constantly compare herself to others" and "measure her self-worth by her likes" her posts received.

Essena said that she had always wanted to become

popular on social media. She kept a close eye on other social media celebrities and tried to act like them to build a following. She posted glamorous shots of herself and her "perfect" life, and she reached her goals. Even though she had hundreds of thousands of followers on Instagram and YouTube, she confessed in one of her videos that instead of finding happiness, social media had consumed her. She was unable to cope with all of the pressure of having to show the perfect life; she shut down some of her channels and changed the others up to show her true self.

Essena was right when she said that social media is not real life. For many, social media is their life. They find their connections, approval, and acceptance through social media. If you went out to dinner with a friend, you don't tell them a story and then ask them to "rate it" or "like it."

This need for validation and approval stems from the innate need to feel included. This is, without a doubt, one of the big reasons why we start using social media. This is especially true when it furthers our sense of belonging or of getting to be a part of something that adds more meaning to our life. While it isn't bad on paper, people must find an environment and community that respects us for what they actually have to offer, for their real accomplishments. This is an attitude that we should all strive to have towards others as well.

Chapter 5: Impact of Social Networks in Our Democracies

Social Networks have been accused of taking over our lives but do they have the ability to take over our government? There have been several instances where other countries have taken control of computers and hacked into people's Facebook and other social media accounts to spread fake news all over the world. We're going to look at a few examples.

Cambridge Analytica

Cambridge Analytica is in the middle of an undercover sting operation where its top executives have been boasting about fake news campaigns, entrapment techniques, and psychological manipulation.

This London-based election consultant along with Facebook is in the middle of a dispute about harvesting and using personal data. These allegations have increased the concerns about where this kind of data got used to influence the Brexit vote outcome and the 2016 United States presidential campaign.

Both of the companies have denied all wrongdoings.

So what happened during the undercover operation? Cambridge Analytica senior executives have been caught on camera, saying they could use misinformation, bribes, and prostitutes to try to help political candidates get votes from all over the world.

They have claimed that the reporter tricked them, and they didn't even have any intention of doing all the things they had talked about.

The reporter from Britain's Channel 4 News was sent in undercover to be a representative of a Sri Lankan family of significant wealth wanting to get some political standing. Even though the executives at first denied that they used "entrapment," after meeting with the reporter several times, they finally told him about some of the tactics that they might use.

This investigation also used articles that were published by the United Kingdom newspaper *The Observer,* along with the *New York Times.* The reports outlined the ways data from millions of Facebook accounts had been shared with Cambridge Analytica

In 2014, Aleksandr Kogan's company Global Science Research developed an app that was called "thisisyourdigitallife." This gave users money to take a psychological test, and the app would collect all of the data that they received. They also took information from the Facebook friends of those who completed the test.

By doing this, they were able to mine 50 million Facebook profiles. Kogan gave Cambridge Analytic his information. This lets the firm build software that was able to influence the choices of voters in various elections.

According to the whistleblower Christopher Wylie, they sold the data to Cambridge Analytica, and they used the psychological profiles of some to send them pro-Trump materials through their Facebook.

They have since denied that they used any of the data to help the Trump campaign.

Facebook's Response

Facebook has stated that even though Cambridge Analytica obtained the information legally, it has claimed that Kogan violated Facebook's policies by lying to the platform because he knew he would be sending all their data to Cambridge Analytica.

In 2015, Facebook banned Kogan's profile and ordered any company that had gotten information from him to destroy all the information. Reports can forth state that the data was never destroyed. Cambridge Analytica has argued repeatedly that it did delete all the information as soon as they were told to.

In a statement released from Facebook: "The entire company is outraged we were deceived. We are committed to vigorously enforcing our policies to protect people's information and will take whatever steps are required to see that this happens."

Facebook also stated that it would have all their senior executives to work continuously to get every fact they could find.

Even though Mark Zuckerberg and Sheryl Sandberg didn't speak publicly about those allegations, they did share some briefs in a congressional committee.

Why This Matters

This story is important due to the way the data was obtained and then used. They used the information to send political messages that Cambridge Analytica supported, and was not used in an unbiased manner. The two elections that seem to be targeted were the Brexit vote and Trump's election.

The role that marketing may have had to do with these campaign outcomes isn't known. Cambridge Analytica has never admitted to any wrongdoing, and probably never will.

One of Cambridge Analytica's executives claimed he spoke with Trump many times and that Analytica was responsible for the majority of his campaign activity during 2016.

He claims: "We did all the research, all the data, all the analytics, all the targeting... We ran all the digital campaigns, the television campaign, and our data informed all the strategy."

He has also stated that he wasn't sure about how accurate all the data the firm had collected was and how it influenced the Trump election.

Russia's Cyberwarfare

Cyberwarfare by Russia does include the persecution of cyber-dissidents, internet surveillance by using SORM technology, participating in political blogs that are run by teams sponsored by the state, circulating propaganda and disinformation, hacker attacks, denying service attacks, among other measures. Some activities were created by the "Russian Signals Intelligence," which is a section of the FSB. One review done by the "Defense

Intelligence Agency" during 2017 said that the Russian view of "Information Countermeasures" as being "strategically decisive and critically important to control its domestic populace and influence adversary states." It would divide the information into two sections; "Informational Psychological" and "Informational Technical." The latter includes operations within networks that relate to exploitation, attack, and defense. The former includes "attempts to change a person's beliefs or behavior in favor of the Russian government's objectives."

Russia's Online Presence

Pete Earley, United States journalist, has described some interviews he had with Sergei Tretyakov, a former intelligence agent. Mr. Tretyakov left Russia for the US in 2000.

He would send somebody to the public library in New York so that they could access the internet without being able to track him. They would then post all kinds of propaganda on different websites and send emails to

US broadcasters and publications. Some of the propaganda was disguised as scientific or educational reports. All the studies were generated by the Center by Russian experts. These reports would always be 100 percent true.

Mr. Tretyakov didn't state the websites that were targeted but made it clear that they selected sites that were the easiest to distribute information. According to Mr. Tretyakov, the most frequent subject during his time in New York was the War in Chechnya.

Cyberattacks

Many companies have stated that the Russian Security Services have formed several "denial of service attacks" as a form of their cyber warfare against other countries. A Russian hacker has stated that the Russian State Security Services paid him to help the country have into NATO computers. When they approached him, he had been studying at the "Department of the Defense of

Information" in computer sciences. The FSB was paying his tuition.

Brexit Referendum

The Brexit referendum referred to the movement when the United wanted to separate from the European Union. David Cameron, Prime Minister, made the comment that Russia would likely be happy if Brexit got a positive vote. The Remain believed that the Kremlin-backed a positive vote. Ben Bradshaw told Parliament in December 2016 that Russia had interfered with the Brexit campaign. Bradshaw contacted the British Intelligence Service, in February 2017, to reveal the information he had about Russian interference.

The Guardian reported in June of 2017 that "Leave" campaigner Nigel Farage was under investigation by the US FBI into the Russian interference in the 2106 US election. In October of 2017, the Parliament demanded that Twitter, Google, Facebook, and other websites to give up all the details and advertisements that Russia had paid for that promoted Brexit.

United States

It was reported that in April 2015, hackers from Russia had "penetrated sensitive parts of the White House computers." The US intelligence agencies, the Secret Service, and the FBI stated that the attacks had been "the most sophisticated attacks that were launched against the US government."

In 2015, CNN had said that Russian hackers had worked for the Russian government in the State Department hack. Members of Congress, intelligence, and federal law enforcement declare the State Department hack the "worst" cyberattack against the federal government

Top Russian cyber official and senior Kremlin advisor, Andrey Krutskikh, in February 2016, told the "Russian National Security Conference" that Russia had been working on new ways to get information that would equal a nuclear bomb test. This would also give them the chance to speak with the United States as an equal.

The emails that had been hacked belonged to Colin Powell, John Podesta, and others who belong to the Democratic National Committee through WikiLeaks and DCLeaks was of Russian origin.

Democrats and Republicans who belonged to the "Senate Committee on Armed Services" asked for a "special committee to investigate Russian attempts to influence the presidential election."

During 2018, the "US Computer Emergency Response Team" sent out a message warning that the Russian government was trying to execute "a multi-stage intrusion campaign by Russian government cyber actions which targeted small commercial facilities' networks where they staged malware, conducted spear phishing, and gained remote access into energy sector networks." They also noted that "after they obtained access, the Russian government cyber actors conducted network reconnaissance, moved laterally, and collected information pertaining to Industrial Control Systems." The hacks had targeted about 12 US power plants, government facilities, aviation, and water processing plants.

Russia's Interference With the 2016 US Elections

Russia's government interfered with the 2016 US election with an end goal of harming Hillary Clinton and boosting Donald Trump. It also wanted to increase the social and political discord within the US. The IRA or Internet Research Agency, located in Saint Petersburg, has been described as being a troll farm. It creates thousands of fake social media accounts that looked to be an American who supports all the radical political groups. It also promoted and planned events to help fund Trump but reported falsely against Clinton. They reached over a million social media accounts between the years 2013 and 2017. Misinformation and false articles were sent from media that was controlled by Russia's government to all the fake social media accounts. Hackers who were part of the GRU or "Russian Military Intelligence Service" hacked into the DCCC, John Podesta (Clinton's campaign official), and DNC's information systems. They also released stolen emails and files from WikiLeaks, Guccifer 2.0, and DCLeaks during the campaign. Many people who are connected to Russia got in contact with different campaign associates of Trumps and offered business deals to the Trump Organization. They also gave them all the damaging information they had on Clinton. All the government officials in Russia have denied all these claims.

This interference triggered statements from American intelligence, closures of some Russian facilities, the firing of their staff, more economic sanctions against Russia, and a warning from President Barack Obama to Vladimir Putin. The House and Senate Intelligence Committees did their own investigation. Trump has denied that any interference happened. He contends that it was a hoax that the Democrats invented to explain why Clinton lost. Trump fired James Comey, the director of the FBI at the time, because of his part in the Russian investigation.

The attempts of Russian's interference with the election were made public by members of Congress on September 22, 2016, and in January 2017, were sent on to the Director of National Intelligence.

According to these agencies, this operation was ordered by Putin. The FBI opened an investigation into Russia's interference on July 31, 2016. It included a focus on links between Russian officials and Trump associates, along with suspected coordination between the Russian government and the Trump campaign. The FBI's work into this matter was taken over by Robert Mueller, who was a former FBI director. He led a "Special Counsel Investigation" until March of 2019. He concluded that all the interference from Russia was systematic and sweeping, and it violated the United States criminal law. He indicted three Russian organizations and 26 Russian citizens. This investigation led to the indictments and conviction of some of Trump's campaign officials and other Americans. Even though Trump's campaign welcomed all the Russian activities and did expect to benefit from them, there wasn't enough evidence to bring any charges against Trump or any of his associates.

Russian's Interference With the US 2018 Elections

The United States Intelligence Community concluded that the Russian government was continuing its interference that it began during the 2016 elections and was trying to influence the 2108 mid-term elections by creating discord through social media. Primaries for certain candidates started in March in some states and continued into September. The leaders of these agencies have seen Russia spreading misinformation through false social media accounts to divide American society and foster what they call anti-Americanism.

Russia's Interference With the 2016 Brexit Referendum

This is still investigations happening about the alleged interference of Russia in the Brexit referendum being conducted by the US Senate and several United Kingdom agencies.

Social Media

Russia's interference in the Brexit referendum did so by promoting misinformation through fake state-sponsored media platforms and social media accounts. In addition to all the interference of the US election of 2016, they have documented Russian trolls promoting fake claims about election fraud and trying to amplify the impact of terrorist attacks. They planted fake photoshopped images and stories trying to create discord in the West and undermining several institutions.

RT

One of the reports from the US Senate stated that RT, a Russian media channel that shared information about the campaign and only gave a one-sided view of the story. A look into this misinformation and fake news that they shared estimated the value of the anti-EU Russian state media that was shared during the Brexit referendum was between 1.4 and 4.14 million £.

Twitter Bots

There was information released by Twitter in 2018 that found 3 841 accounts that originated in Russia that was connected to the "Internet Research Agency," along with 770 accounts that were possibly in Iran. They sent over ten million tweets trying to spread discord and misinformation with a 24 hours blitz during the day when the referendum vote was supposed to be held. There was a study that found 1.5 million tweets contained a hashtag that was connected to the referendum and discovered that a third of every tweet was generated by one percent of the 300,000 samples. They also discovered that they came from pro-remain and pro-leave bots did exist, but the majority of the hashtags were pro-leave.

The Times reported the researchers from UC Berkeley and Swansea University found about 150,000 accounts connected to Russia that had shared tweets about Brexit. Other researchers had documented about 13,493 accounts had tweeted about the Brexit would disappear from Twitter right after the ballot was over.

An analysis from F-secure found that "suspicious activity" related to Brexit posts continued well into 2019. He claimed the activity patterns matched up with the tactics used by the Russian troll farms

Arron Banks' Funding

One of the biggest donors for the Brexit campaign was Arron Banks. Before these donations, Southern Rock, the underwriting company for Banks, was insolvent and required £60m. It received a £77m injection from a company called ICS Risk Solutions. When Rebecca Pow questioned the company, "Banks implied that this was simply him shuffling money between two companies that he owned." Even though Banks states he owns 90 percent of the company, he actually owns between 50 and 75 percent according to files that suggest there might be some undeclared shareholders.

Around this time, Banks and Andy Wigmore began to have meetings with a Russian official in London at the Russian embassy. He had also been seen in Russia trying to raise funds about this same time.

Only a few months after this cash deposit, he began to make huge donations to different political groups, including the £8m for the Brexit campaign.

Russian's Intelligence Agencies Send Misinformation About

COVID-19

Several Russian intelligence agencies have spread misinformation about the COVID-19 pandemic. Material that shows how Moscow has continued to influence American's views as the 2020 presidential election grows near.

GRU, a Russian military intelligence agency, has used InfoRos among other websites to push through propaganda and misinformation about the coronavirus pandemic like amplifying fake Chinese information about the virus having been formed by the US military and articles that have said that assistance from Russia's doctors could bring strained relations to Washington.

These misinformation efforts are more refined than what they did in 2016. The bots and fake accounts that the Internet Research Agency uses to push out this fake information is quite is to remove, but what is hard to do is to stop the circulation of the articles that should up on legitimate-looking websites.

Laura Rosenberger, who is the director at the Alliance for Securing Democracy, states: "Russian intelligence agencies are taking a more central role in disinformation efforts that Russia is pushing now. It is not the blunt force of the operations mounted by the Internet Research Agency."

Two American officials have found newly declassified intelligence, but they won't give up any reports about the SVU and the GRU activity. These are equal to America's CIA. They talked about the information if they could remain anonymous.

There are intelligence officials who have warned about the interference of Iranian, Russian, and Chinese efforts in the 2020 election. Democrats want more specifics, and these officials have promised to give more information later.

Even though the misinformation that was outlined by the official is focused on the pandemic, some researchers have stated that Russia has continued to share false information on various topics.

A part of the FireEye security firm, "Mandiant Threat Intelligence," has reported that it detected another campaign in Eastern Europe trying to discredit the "North Atlantic Treaty Organization," which includes sharing false information concerning the pandemic. Even though they didn't specifically name Russia, it did state the campaign "was aligned with Russian security interests" trying to undermine the activity by NATO

Facebook has actually started to label any story that is shared by news sites like Sputnik and RT. It is more difficult for social sites to label any article that is shared on conspiracy sites.

Most of these pieces that are created by Russian intelligence get published on One World.Press and InfoRos. The Russian government controls both of these sites. There are other sites like GlobalResearch.ca that amplify GRU propaganda on a regular basis. Officials haven't yet linked it to Russian intelligence.

US government has described false information that focuses on the pandemic. They have also found ties between a think tank and the Russian intelligence that has published some stories about politics.

"The Strategic Culture Foundation" is also controlled by the Russian agency SVR. This foundation has ties to Russian intelligence and is being investigated. An article that was published in May by this foundation was very critical of Evelyn Farkas. She was part of the Obama administration and had been running for Congress in New York.

She states that the Russians are repeating their efforts to influence this election just like they did back in 2015. She states: "They want to sow dissent and reduce confidence among Americans in our democracy and make democracy look bad throughout the world. They want to prevent people who are tough on Russia from coming into power."

After this article was published, OneWorld.Press gave a statement that said any type of accusation that stated they had been working with Russian was "categorically false." It went on to say: "to the best of our knowledge," any of the contributors had not been charged with any crime for working with a foreign agency.

Without any sort of evidence, OneWorld.Press stated that all accusations about the propaganda efforts of Russia had been spread by those who are trying to hurt the chances of Trump getting reelected. They stated: "Everybody across the world knows that some members of the deep state have their daggers out for Trump, and the president himself has even said as much on countless occasions."

American officials have said the GRU's psychological warfare team, also called Unit 54777, was the backing group for the propaganda campaigns that tried to hide Moscow's role. One article in *The Washington Post* connected InfoRos to Unit 54777.

The United States has identified two Russians, Aleksandr G. Starunskiy and Denis V. Tyurin, who have ties to the GRU. These men make sure all the false information and messages that get created through the intelligence officials are shared through InfoRos and on OneWorld.Press, as well as InfoBrics.org.

Mr. Starunskiy and Mr. Tyurin were involved in a type of information laundering that is somewhat close to money laundering. They gather up all of the messages that come from Russian intelligence and then share them with OnePress, InfoRos, or other websites.

All of this information gets created by GRU and then is grabbed up by other sites that share it further across the internet. These tend to be on the sidelines of the web, but some, such as Global Research, have strong followings.

Any story that gets pushed by Russian intelligence looks like native English speakers have written them, and they do not stand out in any way as a product of a foreign group.

From around the end of May until the early part of July, around 150 articles concerning the pandemic were shared by the Russian government. OneWorld shares a lot of stories about how the pandemic was simply an experiment to manipulate the world. Tass and InfoRos published one that said the US was using the coronavirus as a way to impose its views on the world.

InfoBrics.org shared a story stating that Bejing said that the coronavirus was a biological weapon that the US had created.

Even though the specific sites might not receive a lot of traffic, but officials think all the false information that gets created by the Russian intelligence groups is intentionally amplified.

Tracking all the influences of the false information sent by Russia is hard. Even though documents that were stolen and then published by Russia played a big role in the 2016 presidential campaign, but false information and propaganda that gets shared on different news sites, such as Global Research or OneWorld, might have a lot more traction.

The things that GRU posts on social media sites normally flop, but the content they write gets shared a lot broader through the niche ecosystem.

Mandiant called their group "Ghostwriter," because they completely relied on fake quotations, letters, or articles that looked like they came from military officials or politicians. They relied on the stories that had been created by what they referred to as "at least 14 inauthentic personas." This means that the group created the blog writers and reporters. The articles were published by sites like TheDuran.com, which is pro-Russian. The American intelligence groups have been looking into these groups as well.

One example is a fabricated letter that looks like it was written by Jens Stoltenberg, the secretary-general at NATO, who kept the false claim that the alliance was going to leave Lithuania when the pandemic began to spread. Another article involved a Lithuanian news site that got hacked, and the hackers posted articles that claimed German troops had desecrated a Jewish cemetery.

Coronavirus False Information and Ways Scientists Can Fight It

Injecting disinfectant or eating sea lettuce isn't going to keep you from getting COVID-19. You can't test for COVID-19 by keeping your breath held for ten seconds. Vladimir Putin didn't release 500 lions in Moscow in order to make residents stay inside to help fight the virus. The spread of COVID-19 has come along with what has been called an infodemic by the WHO. The demand for more information concerning the disease has taken its toll on our lives and the health care system, and all of our unanswered questions have formed a breeding ground for fake news, conspiracy theories, and myths. Some of these can easily be dismissed as ludicrous and pretty much harmless, but some of them can harm lives.

Scientists have the right to fight back against all the false information about COVID-19 but do they need to get involved in all the time-consuming efforts or just continue doing research? For the people who have signed up to fight it, how can all this false information be stopped? Do scientists need to restrict the intervention to what they are experienced in? Is responding to all the falsehoods about COVID-19 a public service, or could there be a career in it?

If scientists are comfortable being on the front line, they could counter all this false information about COVID-19 and help policymakers stay away from making policies that could be harmful, improve the public's understanding of the pandemic, and save countless lives.

The main change that COVID-19 has brought about is how much news gets consumed. One survey looked at 13 countries in March, and it found that because of the pandemic, about 67 percent of the people surveyed watched more news than they used to. Most people refresh their web browsers a lot more now. They are looking for new or more information about the pandemic since it affects our health and the health of families and friends. This makes it more likely for us to get tricked.

Jevin West is a co-creator of a course that is meant to help us spot false statistical and scientific evidence called Calling Bullshit. In December, he became the director of his university's "Center for an Informed Public." It researches rumors and false information during a crisis. They have been busy for several months for them. West states: "It's been all-consuming, a bit like trying to build a boat while you're floating along in the sea."

The False Information World

People looking to minimize harm focuses their time on identifying false medical claims. Researchers located at the "Taiwan FactCheck Center," since the end of January 2020, have spent the majority of their time debunking claims about false tests and remedies. Some involved smelling certain plant oils, cleaning the inside of the nostril with salt water, or breathing in steam can kill COVID-19 before it gets to our lungs. All of this fake information about how to kill this virus comes from the gaps in knowledge surrounding the virus.

The people who share all the myths have just been

misguided but other people who are looking to make money. In March 2020, the USFDA warned individuals and companies like Jim Bakker and Alex Jones to stop selling the benefits of colloidal silver. These two people have sold and promoted products that contain small particles of silver that were suspended in liquid even though there wasn't any evidence about them working to prevent the disease. Another way to make money from false news is through advertising. Around half of all of this false information is from people who are trying to produce content that will get clicked on and then directs people to a website that is nothing Google ads.

Most myths around COVID-19 have a lot of political motivation behind them, like the stories that the virus escaped a Wuhan science lab or was made to be a bioweapon. One survey done in the US in the middle of March found that only six percent believed that virus was accidentally created in a lab and 23 percent hat it was intentionally created. These reports have tried to be debunked along with those that suggest the virus originated in the US and was taken into China.

Scientists could have a stronger impact when controlling these myths that don't have to do with politics. The best way to do this is to make their expertise available to fact-checkers and journalists who debunk false information.

Do scientists need to try to counter all this false information across every field or just stick with their own? The debate about if researchers need to "stay in their lane" had turned into a big discussion during all of this.

Friendly Fire

An intervention's tone determines how it is going to be received. Kerry Katona, a British television personality and singer, shared a post on Instagram that stated children who tested positive with COVID-19 needed to be taken away from their family and put in a hospital by themselves. Ranjit Singh, a British television presenter, and the doctor responded with: "Not true! Facts are facts! I've seen lots of confusion and misinformation about kids and #coronavirus recently." He also shared a list of factual information. Katona thanked him for this and said that it made her feel better. Zagni says we need to stay away from appearing patronizing or confrontational is the key when looking to change a person's mind. We need to have honest discussions with people about why they decided to share certain materials. People should not talk down to others or treat them as if they are stupid. A lot of people out there are simply looking for the truth.

Reminding somebody about the facts that avoids direct confrontations will likely be more effective. There is a study by Gordon Pennycook, a psychologist, that showed two groups from the US various headlines concerning COVID-19. Some of what they saw was false, and some were true, and the participants weren't told which was right. In the first group, about 43 percent of the false headlines and 47 percent of the true headlines were worth sharing. In the next group, they were asked to rate how accurate one headline was that it was not related to COVID-19. This made them a bit more discerning since they said they would share 50 percent of the reports that were true, and 40 percent of those that were false.

Most of the participants found that they were inspired by this and wanted to help contribute to protecting people from false claims to help to lessen the loss of health and life. There might be benefits of getting involved in defending the truth.

Even though being known as a science defender may have some career benefits, there are also some downsides. West states: "It can help professionally, especially for early-career researchers, but it can also take up days and weeks, and it can be hard to return to your own research once you've gotten sucked in." He stated that scientists need to make sure that they don't allow their professional views to help them decide whether or not to help the battle against coronavirus false information. It really shouldn't matter because all lives matter. You have to trust in science. Lives are on the line, and something needs to be done about all of the losses we have incurred.

Chapter 6: Digital Minimalism and Digital Detox

As I am sure you have realized, we all must take a step away from social media and the digital world with a detox. This is how we can keep ourselves sane in our hyperconnected world. We need to adopt sustainable and healthy habits around how we use tech so that we have control over it, and it doesn't control us.

From our pinging watches to digging texts and endless Instagram feeds, we can't deny that we are way more plugged in than we should be. Sure, being connected comes with its benefits. It's a great way to stay in touch with people we don't get to see that often. You are also free to share your opinions, and it can help with multitasking, but we can't ignore its serious drawbacks. If you still aren't sure about taking a break from social media, it has helped our attention span drop from 12 seconds to only eight seconds. We have shorter attention spans than the goldfish. Not only that, but it can create stress. This can translate to neck pain, wrinkles, and high blood pressure.

But it's simply not practical to give up screen time altogether. Thankfully, experts have agreed that you don't need to through your phone out; you simply need to loosen your grip a bit. That's what we're getting ready to discuss.

10-Steps to a Digital Detox

Why should you fool with a digital detox, anyway? Let's assume that you are addicted to social media. Is it really harming anybody? You may still be doing well in school or getting all of your work done at the office. You make sure to take care of yourself and regularly exercise. It isn't like you're addicted to heroin, right?

That is very true, with all things considered. It is likely one of the safest addictions a person could have. Nobody has ever died from it. But how is your quality of life?

Ten-steps, that's not too much to do, is it? Maybe not, but sticking to an actual detox can be difficult. Despite the fact that dopamine is involved, social media addiction is a psychological addiction, just like video game addiction. When it comes to substance-related addictions, there is a gradual weaning process that has to happen because of the physical withdrawal symptoms. With psychological dependence, it is best to deal with it cold-turkey.

Basically, you have to stop rewarding your dopamine triggers so that the brain is able to go back to normal. This can't be done if you are feeding that appetite from time to time. You are also more likely to spiral back into your addiction with small hits. I promised 10-steps, though, so here are those 10-steps that are better done all at once than slowly.

1.   Switch off Push Notifications

Constantly receiving updates on the goings-on in the world is informative, but it also creates a huge distraction. If you are constantly getting distracted, then you aren't going to get anything done. The best way to stop this is to turn off your notifications, or at least as many as you can stand to be without.

2.   Change to Gray Scale

All of the colors on our devices is a big reason why they are attractive. Take things back a few decades and go retro. There are a lot of smartphones that give you the option to place your phone into grayscale.

3.   Put it Up While Eating

Look around a restaurant, and you will likely see at least

one phone out at each table. Whether they are actively using it or not, simply having it out will reduce the quality of the conversation. The brain is waiting to see the phone light up, so we aren't fully present in the moment. The more energy we give our devices, the less we are giving to whoever we are spending time with. If we can't see it, we don't think about it.

4.   Pick Some Tech-Free Hours

People who don't have their phone often feel naked, but taking a bit of a break from technology during the day can do great things. Start by specifying certain hours during a day that will be completely tech-free, such as during your lunch break. After a week, see how you feel with that tech-free time. Most people end up feeling happy about the change, and then they start to expand it.

5.   Bedroom is Tech-Free

A lot of people will use their phones as an alarm clock,

but when you reach up to turn off the alarm, it's easy just to start looking through your various accounts. It's better if you don't allow your phone to come into your bedroom at night at all, and just get a real alarm clock. Plus, if you tend to spend a lot of time on you, you are less likely to spend time with your partner. Make your bed a device-free area so that you have a better chance for sex and intimacy. You will also end up getting better sleep. The blue light that comes from your phone tricks the brain into thinking its daytime, which makes it harder to go to sleep.

6.   Meet Paper, Again

If you have found that reading and the actual book feels better than swiping on a tablet, you aren't imaging things. Books not only have fewer distractions, but there is research that has found that when you read on paper, the mind processes information more efficiently. You should also think about getting news from the newspaper.

7.   Use One Screen At a Time

If you are trying to work, and you start to scroll through your Twitter feed, the brain will go a little haywire. Multitasking is not helpful in any way. If you are working on something and then you get distracted by something, such as, I'll just click onto this new window or check my text message real quick, it is going to take your brain several minutes to return back to what you were originally doing. Make it a habit to only use one screen at a time to make sure that you stay concentrated, and it will improve your enjoyment.

8.   Spring Clean Social Media

Instagram and Facebook help us to connect with people in a way that has never been seen before. Research has found that the more we are on social media, the worse we feel. It's really not all that surprising, considering the fact that we see this strongly built façade, which fosters toxic levels of self-esteem. How can we be on social media and not let it destroy our mental wellbeing?

The key here is to be proactive in your use and about who and what you follow. From that point on, you need to go through and clean the house. Delete, unfollow, mute, or block anybody who is sharing things that makes you feel bad. Come up with a list of friends and celebrities that make you laugh and smile and helps you feel worthy and happy.

9.   Choose The Right Apps

There are plenty of people who feel they are addicted to their phone, and for a good reason. As we know, we get a dopamine release each time we check our phones. While it may not make sense at first, but the types of apps you choose can help you reduce the amount of time you use your phone. The Moment app will track the amount of time you spend on your phone and will help you to set daily limits. Freedom app blocks sites on your computer or devices that may distract you so that you can improve your focus. Off-Time is an Android app that helps you selectively block calls, notifications, and text. Using the "Do Not Disturb" setting on iPhones will do the same thing.

10.   Protect Your Body

The time that the average American spends staring at screens is nearly half a day, and the body can pay a large price for this. To make sure you don't strain your eyes, which can end up causing blurred vision, headaches, and dryness, try the 20-20-20 rule. For every 20 minutes of screen time, look up and at something that is 20 feet aware from you for 20 seconds. Make sure you blink as well while staring at the screen. To make sure you don't get, or to fix, "text neck," stop bending your neck to look at your phone and raise your phone up so that you look straight at it. Make sure you avoid "smartphone thumb," which is a perma-bent texting position that can create inflammation, pain, and irritation, by changing up which fingers you use and take a break from texting.

With these 10-steps in mind, we can look at how to do a deeper social media detox. This is an extreme detox, so to speak, as you will be giving up social media altogether for a certain length of time. While it may be scary to think about giving up social media altogether, even if it is only for a few days, it has a lot of benefits. First off, you'll notice that it will help to clear your mind. We get sucked into this fake world of filters, influences, and models, and all of their posts are just to spark an emotional reaction. Just think about how much better you will use your mental energy and time when you could do things you actually care about. Of course, that's not a real answer as to what the benefits are, so here are some real benefits to taking a break from social media.

1.   More Free Time

When the detox starts out, you will find that you are bored. That compulsion to open Instagram or TikTok whenever you have your phone in hand is going to need to be replaced. You are going to have to use all of the time you spent on your phone doing something else. Hopefully, whatever you decide to do will be more productive.

If you kept yourself in the know through social media, instead of reading about the things you are passionate about, get out there and take action by doing something. If you used social media to stay in touch with your friends, write them a letter or go out with them and spend real time with them.

2.   Less Anxiety

What is inevitably going to happen after about a week or so is that you are going to get rid of a lot of mental clutter? You won't find yourself worrying all day about the headlines or trying out the latest trend. With enough time away from social media, you will find that you are more positive since social media tends to jade us. You will no longer compare yourself. You no longer feel as if you need to keep up. This will result in less anxiety.

3.   Better Mornings

The majority of people like to check their phones as soon as they get up, and some will open up their social media accounts upon waking. They notice a notification, and they have to see what it is. This will end up setting the tone for the rest of the morning, and sometimes for the entire day.

Intentionally avoiding social media will force you to use your time first thing the mornings, either during your commute or your first cup of coffee, in a different manner. Instead of reading a rant on Facebook, read a book. Instead of taking a photo of your breakfast for Instagram, enjoy your breakfast. Instead of seeing what somebody Tweeted, take a walk.

4.   More Mindfulness

You will find that you become more mindful when you don't have social media to distract you. You may notice that during certain times of the day, you start to reach for your phone or type in the URL for your favorite social app. Now, you will be able to stop yourself because you are more mindful of those habits. You'll soon realize just how much mental space and time you had been wasting on those apps. This will help you to be more mindful in your daily routine and activities. It will force you to be present in your day.

When you decide to do your detox, you can choose how long it is going to last, but we'll discuss what research has suggested is the best option in a moment. First, here is what you will need to do for a full detox.

1. Let People Know

The first thing you should do is let people know you are taking a social media detox. Let those with who you interact with the most know that you are going to be offline for a while. This will accomplish a couple of things. First, it is going to keep you accountable. If you are back on in just a few days, those who you told will hopefully call you out. This is going to help you stick to your detox. Secondly, it is also going to let the important people in your life know that you didn't just disappear. There's no sense in telling everybody because most aren't going to notice. Don't take that personally, though. It has nothing to do with you.

2. Deactivate Your Accounts

This is going to serve as a hedge against the need to check on your accounts on a whim, and it's also going to let your friends know that you are away. Most social media accounts will allow you to deactivate the account for a while.

3. Uninstall The Apps

This is going to get rid of any notifications or alerts that you get from the apps, which plays a massive role in your addiction. You won't be able to simply pop onto one of the apps in moments of stillness or boredom. This one and the next are absolutely non-negotiable and required. I can promise you that you will not succeed for even a day if you keep the apps on your phone, or you are going to try to rationalize to yourself that you are only going to check the app once a week.

For your detox to work, you will have to disconnect entirely. If that scares you too much, then make your detox shorter.

4. Block Social Media Sites

This goes for tablets, computers, and laptops. Use some sort of web filtering tool that will restrict your access to social media. A good tool to use is K9 Web Protection. You can also go to the extreme and place OpenDNS on your router, where it blocks these sites for all of the devices connected to it.

5. Replace Social Media with Something Else

It's not good enough to simply excise social media from your life. You need to make sure that you fill that space with something else. Otherwise, you are going to end up finding yourself clawing your way back to your social media accounts. A good way to spend your time is to learn a new skill. Some things you can do is read, spend time with friends and family, learn something new, work on a side project, exercise, or travel. You could also give meditation a shot.

Now, back to how long this detox should last. While there aren't that many studies on the subject, there are plenty of experts who say that it takes about 100 days for dopamine levels to go back to normal levels. It could take longer, depending on how intensely or how long you have been addicted, so you shouldn't be surprised if it takes longer. You don't have to take it to that extreme if you don't feel like you need to. The important part is that you give your brain the chance to rest and reset from excessive social media use.

You may also be wondering if you really do need a digital detox. If the thought has crossed your mind that you may be addicted, then you probably do need a break. If you have ever felt that social media is taking over your life, if it is always on your mind, or if you habitually check your phone, then there is a good chance that you need a break. The detox doesn't need to be forever, and technology does serve a purpose in our lives; you may decide that after a few months away from social media, you don't feel the need to go back.

Now, there is one big objection people often have with giving up social media, and that's missing out on things. This sense of FOMO is a strong one. For some, social media is how they keep up-to-date on everything. For others, it's how they stay in touch with their colleagues, family, and friends. Suppose you feel as if you are going to be out of the loop when it comes to news, don't. If there is something important that happens, you are going to hear it at work or through a family member or friend. Plus, most of the information that you are consuming isn't informing you of anything. It is simply distracting you.

Even if most of the accounts you follow are inspirational, you can find that same inspiration through podcasts, documentaries, and books. Finally, when it comes to staying in touch with others, we could all learn how to put in some more effect. You can email people like we use to have to, or you can write an actual handwritten letter to people. You can also use your phone for what it was originally made for, to call somebody. If all else fails, try to spend more time with your family and friends in person. Sure, people are busy but make an effort, reach out, and you might be surprised.

Quitting Social Media

We have added more and more technology into our lives for various reasons, then we woke up and found that they had become the core of our very existence.

The thing that causes us to feel uncomfortable is feeling as if we are losing control. The majority of people who struggle with a technology addiction aren't stupid or weak

Everyone seems to have stumbled into a digital life that no one signed up for. It might even be more appropriate to say that technology companies and large conglomerates pushed us into it.

Until just recently, everyone assumed that being addicted just applied to drugs or alcohol but more and more evidence shows that behavioral addictions can resemble substance addictions.

The concept of social media, where you post content and then wait for the feedback to come in, is the foundation of the service. Our brains categorize ignoring any kind of new notification as equivalent to snubbing a member of our tribe who wants your attention, which is dangerous to do. That's why we have to fight so hard not to get drug into the addiction. These strategies have to be custom-built. One way to go is through digital minimalism.

Digital Minimalism

These subjects have become all too common in the technology world. You have realized that your relationship with all your digital tools has gotten too overwhelming. You get alarmed and decide to deploy some clever life hacks, and then they report that things have gotten better.

Of all of the underlying behaviors that we would like to fix have been ingrained into us through our parents and social group. These have been backed by psychological mechanisms that provide us with a base instinct of power.

Even if some new form of technology promises to provide us with some kind of support, it is going to have passed some strict tests. Would this be the best way to use technology to support the things we believe in? This will contrast sharply from what a lot of people use as a default. With this mindset, you will be able to choose the technology that you actually like.

Minimalists aren't worried about missing out on things. The things that they are more worried about is diminishing the things that they understand is going to make a great life better.

Digital Minimalism Principles

Before you begin experimenting with digital minimalism, look at these principles for a better explanation about why it works. There are three main principles:

- Clutter is costly

When you clutter your attention and time with too many services, apps, and devices can create a negative cost that could take over all the little benefits that every item gives while in isolation.

- Optimization Is Very Important

In order to get all of its benefits, you have to think carefully about ways you will use your technology.

- Intentionality Can Be Satisfying

People who try to live a minimalist digital life get their satisfaction from a commitment to be more intentional about the way they use their technology.

Thoreau's New Economics

In the book *Walden*, Henry David Thoreau establishes this theory of the following principle. He says: "The cost of a thing is the amount of what I will call life which is required to be exchanged for it, immediately or in the long run."

When a person thinks about adding a certain behavior or tool into their life, they usually focus on just the value that it will produce. Standard thinking tells us the profit from the action is great and that the more you get from it, the better. It starts to make sense that the more digital items you have in your life, the better things will be. This new economics by Thoreau demands that you have to balance the profit with the cost that can be measure by your life.

The Return Curve

You could apply the "Law of Diminishing Returns" in numerous ways when it comes to new technology adding more value to our life. Most people's technology use lies within the return of the curve. This is the area in which all other attempts to optimize will only bring bigger improvements.

If you believe that a service provides you with features that you can put to good use, then you are going to be less likely to use them as often. This is the reason social media platforms are so vague when they describe their platform.

The lesson of An Amish Hacker

Amish people have a tradition where they begin with all the things they value the most and work backward to see if any new technology will bring more harm than good.

They think that intention is better than conventional. This example leaves us with the question of whether or not this value stays even if we get rid of the stricter rules in these communities.

There are excellent reasons to believe in this way. Margaret's satisfaction with her life without a smartphone comes from the choice. She states: "My decision not to use a smartphone gives me a sense of autonomy. I control the role technology plays in my life."

When you outsource your self-government to the conglomerates, it can degrade your individuality.

Digital Declutter

Some people have found that slowly changing our habits doesn't work all that well. It is sometimes best just to rip the band-aid off as fast as possible. The following idea of digital decluttering plays off of the idea of the detox we talked about in the last chapter.

The Process of Decluttering

You need to set aside 30 days where you step away from all technology. When you are on this break, you should explore and try to find all the behaviors and activities that you feel are meaningful and satisfying. When the break is over, you can begin reintroducing some of your optional technologies. Begin from a blank space. For every technology that you bring back into your life, figure out its value and how you will use it so you can maximize its value.

The biggest culprit was that the restriction rules were either too strict or too vague. Another mistake that people were having was that they hadn't been planning what they would replace the technology during this period of decluttering. Those who viewed this as a detox, where all they were doing was taking a break from technology before they headed back to using it like they normally work, also struggled.

Define the Rules

The first thing you need to do is figure out what technology would fall into the decluttering. Reddit, Instagram, Facebook, Twitter, text messages are all examples of the technology that you need to look at when you are getting ready for your digital declutter. Your electric toothbrush, radio, microwave, etc. would not be included.

It helps if you view your technology use as being optional unless removing it would disrupt or harm your daily personal or professional life. Use operating procedures when looking at very optional technology. These procedures will show you exactly when and how you use a certain technology. This will give you the chance to use it when you have to without spiraling out of control again.

30-Day Break

As time goes by, the symptoms of the detox will wear off, and you will start forgetting about the technology. The goal isn't that you are just giving yourself a break, but a permanent change. In order for you to succeed at this, you have to take this time and find the things that you feel are important and find joy in the real world. You need to figure this out before you start bringing technology back into your life.

Bringing Technology Back Into Your Life

This step is a bit more demanding than it might sound. It would be best if you were starting from a blank slate and bringing in technology that passes through your new strict standards. When considering bringing back a digital item, answer these questions for each item:

- How will I use this technology to minimize its harms and maximize its value?

- Is it going to help support my values?

- Does this item support things that I value deeply?

A digital minimalist will fight this by using operating procedures that will let them know how and when they are using certain items. One unique experience that was shared by some friends as they quickly went back to their optional devices just to realize that they no longer enjoyed them.

Practices

Getting Some Alone Time

Solitude has to do with the things going on in your brain and not the things going on around you. You have the ability to enjoy solitude even if you are sitting in a crowded coffee shop, on a train, in a car, or at home, as long as your mind only has to think about its own thoughts.

Solitude can come to an end in the quietest areas if you allow input from someone else's mind to intrude into yours. Solitude means you have to get past that reaction to information that they receive from others and focus solely on your own experiences and thoughts, and it doesn't matter where you are at.

To quote Blaise Pascal: "All of humanity's problems stem from man's inability to sit quietly in a room alone."

Michael Harris, a Canadian social critic, is worried that new technology can make a culture that ends up undermining the time that you spend alone with your thoughts. Solitude presents three main benefits:

- Closeness to other people

- Understanding yourself

- New ideas

When you can calmly experience separation, it can help foster appreciation over your interpersonal connections. Having solitude on a regular basis, combined with our own social standing, is needed to survive.

This solitude is starting to fade away. The iPod gave us the ability to be constantly distracted. The smartphone gave us a technique to get rid of the rest of our moments of solitude.

It is possible to get rid of solitude totally. The average user will spend about three hours each day looking at their phone screen. The average user will pick up their phone about 39 times every day.

Every time you avoid solitude, you miss out on the good things that it can bring to your life: being able to figure out difficult problems, regulating your emotions, building courage, and strengthening relationships.

In one study done in 2015, they found that teenagers were on their phones about nine hours each day, and this included social media and text messages. All of a sudden, more and more people have anxiety or another similar disorder.

This rise of anxiety-type issues happened with the first group of students who grew up on social media and smartphones. Beginning in 2012, there was a big change within the emotional states of teenagers that wasn't gradual. The slopes on a line graph started to become huge cliffs and vertical mountains. The common characteristics that had been seen from the Millennial general started to disappear.

People who were born between 1995 and 2012, a group that is being called iGen, showed some vast differences when compared to the generation that was before them.

The number of teen suicide and depression has skyrocketed in recent years due to an increase in anxiety disorders. Many people just assume teenagers could dismiss all of this as typical parental grouching, but that wasn't the case. Teenagers who were experiencing anxiety agreed 100 percent. The other thing that grew alongside teenage anxiety was how many young people had smartphones.

After an entire group unintentionally got rid of their alone time, their mental health began suffering. The teenagers lost their ability to understand and process their emotions. They weren't able to reflect on what mattered to them and who they really are. They weren't able to build good relationships or give their brains a chance to turn off.

Humans have to have some sort of solitude to thrive. In the past decade or so, without us even realizing what was happening, we have systematically reduced this main ingredient from our lives.

Leave Your Phone

You need to spend time away from your digital devices. In order to be successful at this, you have to get rid of the belief that you have to have your phone on you at all times, or something terrible will happen.

This isn't about getting rid of your phone. You are still going to have your phone with you most of the time to enjoy it. It is trying to show you that you can live a life where you might not always have a phone within arm's reach.

Take Walks

To quote Nietzsche: "Only thoughts reached by walking have value."

Nietzsche took an eight-hour walk each day. He just thought during this time. He filled up six notebooks with his thoughts in the books *The Wanderer and His Shadow.*

The main reason to walk is that it is a great source of solitude. This practice is pretty simple. Take long walks on a regular basis. Try to find a scenic place. You need to walk alone (as long as the place you are walking is in a safe neighborhood). This means that you need to be by yourself without your phone. Again, you need a space where you feel safe and comfortable.

If you wear headphones, monitoring your text messages, or narrating your walk on Instagram, you aren't actually walking.

The hardest thing to do is to make that time for the walk. It will help if you can broaden how you look at "good weather." You can still walk if it is cold, just put on an extra layer of clothing. You can even walk in the snow as long as it isn't too deep. You can even walk in light rain.

I have found that I am a lot more productive and happier when I can walk regularly.

Write Yourself A Letter

Everybody's notebook serves them in different ways. For me, it was a way to write myself letters when I have encountered inspiration, difficult emotions, or hard decisions. By the time I had finished writing out my thoughts, I had usually gained some clarity.

The act of writing is what brings you the benefits. The brain's region that defines the network is identical to the area that is affected through social experiments.

If our brain is given downtime, our brain will begin to think about our social life. When we lose social connections, it triggers the same system as pain. OTC painkillers can reduce social pain.

Social Media Contradiction

If a person receives composed or targeted information that was written by somebody they know, they will feel better. But if they received composed or targeted information from somebody they didn't know, they didn't have a sense of well being.

Research has found that the more often people use

social media, the bigger the chance was they would feel lonely. The results show that using Facebook negatively affected their wellbeing. They found that if you increase the number of clicked links or likes, mental health will decrease between five and eight percent.

Reclaiming Conversations

Here is an example of our connections: the bandwidth interactions that define our online lives.

Here is an example of a conversation: the richer, higher bandwidth communications that define our social lives.

I want you to understand that I am not arguing for no technology. I am advocating for more conversations. It is a sort of philosophy for socializing during this digital age.

Most people think that connection and conversation as two different ways to accomplish the same goal of keeping their social status.

"Conversation-Concentric Communication" argues that conversation is one of the best types of interaction that will help you keep a relationship. Anything sent as a text, or that isn't interactive isn't a real conversation. The connection will become nothing more than a logistics role.

Stop Clicking Like

Stop clicking "like." Quitting leaving comments on everything you see on social media. They are training you to think that having a simple connection is good enough to replace a real conversation. If you can get rid of all these trivial interactions, you are sending your mind a clear message: discussions are all that count.

If you think not leaving comments is going to be noticed, invest the time to create real conversations.

Consolidate Your Texts

Keep your phone on "Do Not Disturb." Schedule certain times for text messages and let your family and

166

friends know these times. If anyone texts you outside of these times, DON'T answer.

If your family and friends have the ability to have small conversations with you throughout the day, it is easier for you to be complacent within the relationship. Not always being there to answer a text can help improve a relationship.

Have Office Hours

Set aside some times during your day when you will be available to talk. Tell the people that you care about so they can still get in touch with you.

A variation of this would be to choose some time every week where you are going to somewhere and let the people in your life known when you will be there. If they want to see you, they can come to this place and talk to you in person.

Reclaim Your Leisure Time

More and more people are not creating good quality leisure time, which is needed for happiness. This makes an unbearable void. This can be ignored by digital noise. If people are given a lot of downtimes, they are going to fill it with some type of strenuous activity likely.

Use Your Skills To Make Valuable Things

Playing games can give you "supercharged socializing interactions" with high levels of intensity that are normal within polite society. Volunteer activities, recreational sports, social fitness, and board games would be good examples of these.

Find Activities that Take Social Interactions

The internet has caused a "leisure renaissance" by allowing us to have a lot more leisure time. It gives people a chance to discover communities that are connected to their interests and gives them a chance to find information that they need to pursue that interest. There is still digital technology involved, but it has been reduced down to a supportive role.

New technology, if you use it with intention and care, is going to make your life better.

Build or Fix Something Weekly

- Begin a garden

- Build some custom furniture

- Take up and instrument or a language

- Install a new light fixture

- Give your car a tune-up

Schedule Low-Quality Leisure

Schedule some time where you can spend it on some low-quality leisure. Don't worry about the amount of time you set aside for this, as most social media users get the most significant value in only 20 to 40 minutes each week. Fill in your free time with some high-quality alternatives.

Tech Could Protect Us

We've talked about how lousy technology can be, but what if I said that it could be more helpful than harmful. With the distracting nature of technology, it often leaves us feeling like it's either all or nothing. We can either stay distracted, connected, and unproductive, or sign-out, log-off, and let FOMO set in.

A former design ethicist at Google, Tristan Harris, believes that this imbalance is calling for a change in design. This change can help to restore choice. It will give us a choice over our relationship with technology and how we spend our time. However, to accomplish this, we have to find tech companies who make more conscious decisions about their product's goal. Instead of focusing on the metrics of efficiency, users, shares, likes, matches, and so on, companies need to start measuring success through meaningful metrics. These metrics would seek to measure net positive contributions to life.

For example, what if social networks looked for success based on how many jobs offer people received that they liked, instead of the more typical metrics of how many connections were made and messages sent. It is through concerns and conversations like these that can help to start building a world of technology that actually works for us instead of the other way around. This change could create a world where we don't just spend our time, but spend it well.

Conclusion

Thank you for finishing the book, and I hope that you have found all of it informative and helpful. I hope that you have learned how to cut back on your digital dependency and can take your life into your own hands.

The next step is to start evaluating your digital life. Have you been using social media as a way to escape life? Do you allow the internet and all of its bells and whistles to control your life and keep you from doing what you should? These are the questions that you need to answer and exam to figure out how you should proceed.

Social media and the internet is always going to be there, and it's fine to use them, but within reason. Addiction to social media is very real. It causes the release of dopamine, just like any other drug. If you are one of the lucky few to become famous on social media, then the urge to constantly be on there and make your followers happy is stronger. You must find a healthy balance between your real-life and your online life.

Accepting the fact that the digital world isn't healthy and that there are people who use it to manipulate others simply isn't an easy thing to process. For those who have grown up with the internet, or even grown with the internet, it's crazy to think it could be so bad. But with the information you have learned, you can move forward with the caution and curiosity that we all need to have when dealing with the digital world. This will help put us at arm's length so that we don't end up getting taken advantage of or experience any ill-effects.

By acknowledging the risks of the internet and all that is there, you can start to notice possible problems. That's is the first step in making sure you don't get an addict, and you don't allow yourself to be ruled by your digital life. Take a digital detox, and see how it feels. You'll find that you don't need the digital world as much as you think yours do. You'll start feeling better you will be in control of your life once more.

Finally, if you found this book useful in any way, a review on Amazon is always appreciated!

Made in the USA
Middletown, DE
07 November 2020